Five Patients

FIVE
PATIENTS

The Hospital
Explained

Michael Crichton

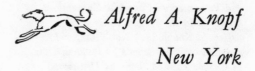 *Alfred A. Knopf*
New York

FOR *Joan*

WHO KNOWS HOW IT WAS

Doctors and nurses are the only people who possibly can alter the conditions of patient care.

PAUL B. BEESON, M.D.

Health, as a vast societal enterprise, is too important to be solely the concern of the providers of services.

WILLIAM L. KISSICK, M.D.

Foreword

There has recently been a lot of foolish talk about something called "the new medicine." To the extent that it implies a distinction from some form of old medicine, the phrase has no meaning at all. Medicine has crossed no watershed; there has been no triumphant breakthrough, no quantum jump in science or technology or social application.

Yet there is, within medicine itself, a sense that things are different. It is difficult to define, for it is not the consequence of change, but rather the fact of change itself.

The first time I began to look at the Massachusetts General Hospital in the spring of 1969 I had the uneasy feeling there was too much flux, too much instability in the system. I felt a little like an interviewer who has come upon his subject at a bad time. Only later did I realize that there would never be a "good" time, and that change is a constant feature of the hospital environment. The true figurehead of modern medicine is not Hippocrates but Heraclitus.

To trace a history of change, one must go back about fifty years, to the time when organized research began to produce major new scientific and technological advances. Medicine has been revolutionized by those advances, but they have not stopped. Indeed, the pace of change has increased. Within the past ten years, social pressures have been added to those of science and technology, producing a demand for a new concept of medical care, a new ethic of responsibility for the doctor, and a new structuring of institutions to deliver broader and better care.

As a result, medicine has become not a changed profession but a perpetually changing one. There is no longer a sense that one can make a few adjustments and then return to a steady state, for the system will never be stable again. There is nothing permanent except change itself.

From this standpoint, the experiences of five patients in a university teaching hospital are most interesting. It should be stated at once that there is nothing typical about either the patients described here or the hospital in which they were treated. Rather, they are presented because their experiences are indicative of some of the ways medicine is now changing.

These five patients were selected from a larger group of twenty-three, all admitted during the first seven months of 1969. In talking to these patients and their families, I identified myself as a fourth-year medical student writing a book about the hospital. As they are presented here, each patient's name and other identifying characteristics have been changed.

I chose these five from the larger group because I

thought their experiences were in some way particularly interesting or relevant. Accordingly, this is a highly selective and personal book, based on the idiosyncratic observation of one medical student wandering around a large institution, sticking his nose into this room or that, talking to some people and watching others and trying to decide what, if anything, it all means.

M.C.

La Jolla, California
November 15, 1969

Acknowledgments

I am greatly indebted to the employees and medical staff of the Massachusetts General Hospital for a kindness and patience that went beyond any reasonable expectation.

I would also like to thank Drs. Robert Ebert, Hermann Lisco, Joseph Gardella, and Mr. Jerome Pollock, all of the Harvard Medical School, for encouragement and advice in planning the book; Drs. Howard Hiatt, Charles Huggins, Hugh Chandler, Ashby Moncure, James Feeney, Joel Alpert, Edward Shapiro, Josef Fisher, Michael Soper, Jerry Grossman, and Miss Kathleen Dwyer for their suggestions at various points in my work; Drs. Alexander Leaf, Martin Nathan, Jonas Salk, and Mr. Martin Bander for their review of the manuscript at different points; Mr. Robert Gottlieb and Miss Lynn Nesbit for ongoing, tireless work on the project; and finally Dr. John Knowles, whose influence is everywhere in this book, as it is in the hospital he directs. With all this help, the book ought to be flawless, and to the extent that it is not, I am to blame.

The late Alan Gregg once quoted a former teacher as saying, "Whenever you say anything explicitly to anyone, you also say something else implicitly, namely,

that you think you are the guy to say it." Such senti-
ments trouble all but the most egotistical writers; the
others recognize that their sense of enfranchisement is
a gift of the people around them, whom they can only
hope not to disappoint.

Contents

Foreword ix

RALPH ORLANDO

In the early hours of the morning, the Massachusetts General Hospital was notified by Harvard University that some students, at that time occupying a university building in protest of ROTC, might be brought to the hospital for treatment of injuries after their forcible removal from the building. This occurred at 5 a.m., and although some fifty students were reportedly injured, none were brought to the MGH.

At 5:45 in the morning, the last of the emergency-ward residents got to bed, sleeping fully clothed, sprawled on a cot in one of the treatment rooms. Taped on the door to the room was a piece of paper on which he had written his name and "Wake at 6:30." Across the hall in another treatment room, two surgical resi-

3

dents were sleeping; in a third room, one of the interns.

Even without the Harvard students, it had been a busy night. Shortly before midnight, the EW had admitted two college students with pelvic fractures from motorcycle accidents, and both had been taken to surgery; later on, they had also admitted a forty-one-year-old man suffering from a heart attack, an eighty-year-old woman with congestive heart failure, and a thirty-six-year-old alcoholic with acute pancreatitis. An elderly man with metastatic carcinoma and renal failure had died at 3 a.m.

There had also been the usual number of patients with sore throats, coughs, abrasions, lacerations, foreign bodies inhaled or swallowed, bruises, concussions, dislocated shoulders, earaches, headaches, stomachaches, backaches, fractures, sprains, chest pains, and breathing difficulties.

At 6:30, some of the junior residents and interns were up, doing lab studies and checking on the patients who had been admitted for observation to the overnight ward, adjacent to the emergency ward. The ONW limited patients to a three-day stay; it was designed for patients who required a period of observation longer than a few hours, such as those with suspected gastrointestinal bleeding or those with severe concussions. However, in practice it was also used for patients who were severely ill but could not get a bed at the time they arrived, because the hospital was full.

At 7 a.m., surgical rounds were made in the ONW.

Six patients were discussed during half an hour, but most of the time was given over to a fifty-four-year-old woman with a recurrence of bleeding ulcer. This was her second day in the hospital and her condition was now stable; she had received five units of blood the day before. Normally she would not be a surgical candidate, but on two previous admissions she had shown the same pattern of massive, unexpected bleeding, followed by stabilization in the hospital after transfusion. The residents were afraid that if this happened again, she might bleed to death before she got to the hospital.

The emergency-ward residents attended these rounds, for in the early morning the EW is least busy. A short distance away, however, the acute psychiatric service was in full swing. The APS always gets a group of patients in the morning; they are the people who, for one reason or another, have not been able to sleep the previous night.

In one of four interview rooms in the APS, a nineteen-year-old girl, separated from her husband, chain-smoked as she described her unsuccesssful attempts to kill her three-year-old daughter: first by hanging, then by suffocation with a pillow, and finally by gas asphyxiation. She explained that she wanted to stop the child from crying; the crying was driving her crazy. She came to the APS, she said, because "I wanted to talk to somebody. I mean, it's not natural, is it? It's not natural—a kid that keeps crying that way."

In another room, a forty-year-old accountant was running down a list of eight reasons why he had to divorce his wife. He had written out the list so he would be sure to remember everything when he talked to the doctor.

In a third room, a college student living on Beacon Hill explained that she was depressed and troubled by a recurrent sensation that came to her during parties. She said she would have the impression that she was invisible and that she was watching the party from across the room, from a different viewpoint. She had attempted suicide two days before by swallowing a bottle of aspirin tablets, but she had vomited them up.

In the fourth room, a husky fifty-one-year-old construction worker discussed his fear that he was going to die suddenly. He knew the fear was groundless but he could not shake it, and his work was suffering, since he was afraid to exert himself and lift heavy objects. He was also bothered by sleeplessness, irritability, and bad headaches. On questioning it developed that his father had died of a stroke almost exactly six years before; the patient remembered his father as "a cold fish that I never liked."

In the lobby of the APS were three other people waiting to talk to the psychiatrists. One woman was crying softly; another stared vacantly out the window. A middle-aged man in a tuxedo and ruffled shirt smiled reassuringly at everyone else in the room.

✠

At 8:30 in the morning, a sixty-year-old widow arrived in the EW and asked to have a doctor remove her hangnail. The administrators at the front desk shrugged and told her it would cost her fourteen dollars. She insisted it was sufficiently important to warrant the expense. But the triage officer flatly refused to do it and told her to cut it herself. Unsatisfied, she wandered around for another fifteen minutes until she finally cornered a resident. She linked her arm in his and demanded that, since he was such a nice young doctor, he please cut her hangnail. He did; she was billed.

Twenty minutes later, a thirty-five-year-old housewife was brought in by the police after she had collapsed in a subway station and suffered an epileptic fit. Soon thereafter, a desperately ill elderly man with disseminated colonic cancer was transferred in from a nursing home. He had a cardiac arrest in the emergency ward and died shortly before noon.

An eighteen-month-old infant with a skin rash was brought in by his mother at noon. The mother wanted to know if it was German measles; she was pregnant and had never contracted the disease. A diagnosis of German measles was made, but the mother, in her sixth month of pregnancy, was reassured that there was no danger to her.

At approximately the same time, an eighteen-year-old secretary arrived, accompanied by the head of personnel at the office where she worked. The girl had reportedly collapsed after lunch. At the time of her arrival she was conscious, but unwilling or unable to speak. She was placed under observation in a room where she lay curled up in bed, burrowing her head beneath the sheets. Medically, she appeared sound, and a psychiatrist was called. He diagnosed an acute psychotic break. By then, her family and some fellow workers had arrived. All regarded the episode as shocking in its suddenness and repeated the observation that she had never acted unusually in the past. The psychiatrist came away shaking his head.

By 1 p.m., a man with a deep laceration of his index finger had arrived; also a woman with a sore throat; another man with a dislocated finger (a taxi door had slammed on his hand); and an eight-year-old boy brought in by his mother. The child had fallen from his bicycle that morning and struck his head. The mother didn't know whether he had been unconscious or not, but she thought he was acting oddly, and noted that he had refused to eat lunch.

No patients more seriously ill arrived, and the atmosphere in the emergency ward during the afternoon was relaxed. The residents took the chance to take it easy, drink coffee in the doctors' room, and catch up on reports in the charts they had to write.

At 3:40, the atmosphere abruptly changed. The hospital's station at Logan Airport called to report that there had been an accident: a dozen construction workers had been injured and were on their way in police cars and ambulances. At least two of the injured were going to

8

Boston City Hospital; as many as ten might come to the MGH. The extent of injuries was not known, but some might be very severe.

The emergency-ward administrator put out a disaster call, notifying the chiefs of all departments of the impending emergency and its nature. The chiefs in turn arranged for mobilization of all available hospital personnel from other wards. In a matter of minutes, interns, residents, and senior men began to appear in the EW. The nurses and staff were already clearing patients out of the treatment rooms; the corridors were cleared and supply carts checked. Privately, everyone agreed that it was fortunate the day had been a slow one, for there was practically no back-up.

Emergency-ward personnel are always concerned about back-up. The emergency ward is geared to treat a new patient every eight minutes, around the clock; the staff is prepared to admit to the hospital one out of every five of these emergency patients, or a new admission every forty minutes. This is a furious pace, but it is standard procedure for the hospital. And although patient flow through the EW is generally smooth, there is almost always a back-up. At any time—and this day was an exception—the emergency ward may have three to ten people in the lobby waiting to be seen; another six to ten in the various treatment rooms; another four or five in the back room waiting for X rays, orthopedic examinations, or sutures of minor lacerations. This is the back-up, and the residents keep an eye on it; when it begins to swell, everyone worries, because there is no way to predict when there will be a six-car automobile crash, or a fire, or some other disaster that will strain the hospital's facilities for emergency care. It is a little like trying to direct traffic without ever knowing when rush hour will occur.

The first patient from Logan Airport to arrive was Thomas Savio, a twenty-seven-year-old bearded construction worker. He arrived in a state police ambulance and was wheeled in wrapped in a gray wool blanket. He was shivering and had severe facial lacerations.

"There's a worse one coming," one of the troopers said. Moments later, John Conamente arrived, groaning. As his stretcher came through the door, one of the residents asked him what hurt. He said it was his shoulder and his leg. Conamente was followed by Albert Sorono, also on a stretcher, complaining of severe pain in his chest and difficulty in breathing.

By now the waiting room was filled with troopers and policemen. The families of the injured men had not yet begun to arrive. Hospital personnel who had not been informed of the accident but had noticed the cluster of policemen stopped to inquire what was happening. At this time, no one really knew the nature of the accident and there was widespread confusion about it; most people thought an airplane had crashed at Logan. A curious crowd began to gather in the lobby. The EW administrators were busy trying to get identifying information on the patients and also attempting to keep the passageways from becoming clogged. "We got seven more coming," one of them said over and over.

A few minutes later, another ambulance pulled up and Ralph Orlando, a fifty-five-year-old father of four, was taken off. He had suffered a cardiac arrest on the way to the hospital and closed cardiac massage was being given by a nurse, the first person who happened to reach him as he was taken from the ambulance. Orlando was wheeled in at a dead run; the massage was taken over by a resident. The patient was taken to OR 1, where full resuscitative procedures were begun.

The routine of cardiac resuscitation is now so standard that few people realize how recent it is. The basic principle of closed cardiac massage was first properly described in modern times in 1960. (It had been described in the nineteenth century but was not commonly practiced.) Prior to that time, a cardiac arrest was almost certainly fatal. The only treatment was thought to be open massage, in which the surgeon incised the chest and squeezed the heart directly with his fingers. Although frequently successful, open massage rarely produced long-term benefit; one study in 1951 indicated that of patients who underwent open massage, only 1 per cent survived to be discharged from the hospital. That figure still stands; open massage is now a last-ditch effort only.

Closed cardiac massage depends upon the anatomical fact that the heart is tightly packed in the chest between breastbone and backbone. Rhythmic pressure upon the breastbone will squeeze the heart enough to

11

produce a pulse. Direct open massage is therefore not necessary, and the hazards of this surgery are avoided.

The purpose of cardiac massage is to maintain blood circulation which, in conjunction with artificial respiration, provides blood oxygenation for the brain. The brain is the organ most sensitive to lack of oxygen; under most circumstances brain damage will begin after three minutes of circulatory arrest. In contrast, the heart itself is much more durable and can resume beating after ten or more minutes. But by this time, unless resuscitation has already been begun, the brain will be irreversibly damaged.

In some situations, mere compression of the heart is enough to start it beating again, but the massage is generally accompanied by a variety of other maneuvers to correct metabolic changes from the arrest. This includes the injection of adrenalin, calcium, and sodium bicarbonate. The experience of the last decade, utilizing these techniques, has demonstrated that cardiac arrest is reversible to an astonishing extent.

The procedure for Ralph Orlando was the standard one: closed massage and artificial ventilation, with simultaneous injection of substances to correct metabolic imbalance. This procedure failed to induce spontaneous contractions of the heart muscle. Electrical defibrillation was then begun.

No one had any idea how long it had been since Orlando had suffered his arrest; presumably whoever had

12

ridden with him in the ambulance knew, but that person could not be found.

Initial electroshock therapy failed. Using a long needle, adrenalin and calcium were now injected directly into the right heart ventricle, and further shocks were administered. It was now twelve minutes since his arrival.

While this was going on, the rest of the EW staff was organizing itself around the other patients. One resident was assigned to oversee the care of each injured man. In the operating room across from Orlando, John Conamente was also surrounded by people. He was simultaneously being examined by the orthopedic surgeons, having intravenous lines inserted in both arms, having blood samples drawn, being catheterized, and being questioned by the resident, who stood at his head and shouted in order to be heard over the noise of the people working around him. The resident conducted a typically stripped-down history and systems review, which under normal conditions might take ten or twenty minutes.

The resident asked, "What happened? Did it fall on you?" (At this time, most people still did not know the nature of the accident, except that something had fallen on a group of construction workers.)

"Yeah," John Conamente said.

"Where did it hit you?"

"My leg."

"Where else? Did it hit your shoulders?"

"Yeah."

"Did it hit your head?"

"No."

"Were you unconscious?"

"No."

"Does your left arm hurt?"

"Yes."

"Your other arm?"

"No."

"Your right leg hurt?"

"Yes."

"You have pain anywhere else?"

"No."

"Your chest hurt?"

"No."

"Breathe okay?"

"Yes."

"Pain in your belly?"

"No."

"Pain in your back?"

"No."

"You ever been in the hospital before?"

"No."

"You ever had an operation before?"

"No."

"Any heart trouble?"

"No."

"Any trouble with your kidneys?"

"No."

"You allergic to anything?"

"No."

"Can you see me all right?"

"Yes."

The resident held up his hand, fingers spread wide. "How many fingers?"

"Five. I'm thirsty. Can I have a drink?"

"Yes, but not now."

By now the orthopedists had concluded their examination. Conamente had fractures of his left arm and right leg.

Out in the hallway, another group was working on Thomas Savio, who complained of difficulty in breathing, pain in his chest, and pain in his lower abdomen. He had a large bruise over his right hip. There was a possibility of pelvic and rib fractures. A laceration on his forehead, while bleeding profusely, was superficial. He was wheeled off for X rays.

Meanwhile in OR 1, attempts at resuscitation were discontinued on Ralph Orlando. Half an hour had passed since his arrival in the hospital. The resuscitation team filed out to help with the other patients, and the door to the room was closed, leaving behind two nurses to remove the intravenous lines and catheters and drape the body in a sheet.

Out in the lobby, John Lamonte, one of the workers, sat in a wheelchair and described what had happened. He was the least injured of all the men, though he had fallen from a height of thirty-five feet. "We were on a scaffolding," he said, "building an airplane hangar. There were three scaffoldings, all about thirty-five or forty feet up. One of them blew down in the wind. It came down real slow, like a dream. There were about twelve people on it, and some underneath." As he spoke, he gathered a crowd of listeners.

Across the room, one of the administrators was telephoning the City Hospital for a woman, to inquire about her brother-in-law. He had been taken there and not to the General. The woman bit her fingernails and watched the expression of the man telephoning. Finally he hung up and said, "He's fine. Just some lacerations on his hands and face. He's fine."

"Thank God," the woman said.

"If you want to get over there, there are cabs in front."

The woman shook her head. "My husband's here," she said, pointing down to the treatment rooms.

Ralph Orlando was then wheeled out on a stretcher. A woman who had just arrived in the EW for treatment of a rash on her elbows stared at the body. "Is he dead?" she asked. "Is he dead?"

Someone said yes, he was dead.

"Why do they cover up the face that way?" she asked, staring.

In another corner of the room, a woman who had been sitting stolidly with a young child got up and took her child out of the lobby while the body was wheeled out.

The emergency ward then received word that there

would be no more people coming, that it would get no more than the six it already had. By now equilibrium was returning to the ward. People were no longer running and there was a sense that things were in control. The state troopers had for the most part gone, but the relatives were still arriving.

Mrs. Orlando, a stout woman accompanied by two teen-age children, was one of the many who immediately tried to leave the lobby and get back to the treatment rooms. All relatives were being prevented from doing this, because the area around the patients was already badly crowded with hospital personnel. Mrs. Orlando was insistent, however, and the more resistance she met, the more insistent she became. The EW administrators tried to coax her out of the lobby and into a more private waiting room. She demanded to see her husband immediately. She was then told that he was dead.

She seemed to shrink, her body curling down on itself, and then she screamed. Her daughter began to sob; her son tearfully swung at members of the staff, his arms arcing blindly. After a moment of this, he began to pound and kick the wall and then, following the example of his sister, he tried to comfort his mother. Mrs. Orlando was crying, "No, no, I won't let you say that." She allowed herself to be led into another room. There was a short silence, and then she cried loudly. Her sobs were heard in the lobby for the next hour.

An MIT undergraduate, working in the emergency

ward on a computer study project, watched it all. "I don't know how anybody can stand to work here," he said.

Dr. Martin Nathan, a surgical resident who had also seen it, said to him, "There are good ways to find out, and there are bad ways to find out. That was a bad way."

"Are there any good ways?" the student asked.

"Yes," the resident said. "There are."

A few minutes later, a nurse went into the private room with sedation for Mrs. Orlando and her family. Soon thereafter, the emergency ward received confirmation that the remaining casualties had been treated at other hospitals. The five in the emergency ward were being cared for; three would go to surgery in the next hour. The extra personnel began to leave, in twos and threes, and things slowly returned to normal. One hour and ten minutes had passed since the first patient arrived.

At 6 p.m., a forty-six-year-old insurance salesman arrived after vomiting up blood; twenty minutes after that, a man came in with his sixty-one-year-old mother, who had suddenly lost her ability to speak and seemed to have trouble keeping her balance; then came a nineteen-year-old graduate student who had broken a glass while washing dishes and cut her ankle. At 7 p.m. arrived a thirteen-year-old boy who had been sideswiped by a car and had suffered a scalp laceration. At seven thirty, a child who had fallen out of bed and cut his forehead; at eight, a fifty-year-old man suffering from a heart attack; moments later, an unresponsive twenty-year-old girl who had swallowed a bottle of sleeping pills, brought in by her roommates; a two-year-old child who cried and tugged at his ear; a nineteen-year-old boy with appendicitis; a thirty-six-year-old woman who had driven her car into a telephone pole and was unconscious; a fifty-nine-year-old alcoholic who said he had been beaten by two sailors and had facial lacerations; a man who was thought to be in a diabetic coma; a linotype operator who had burned his left hand; an elderly man who had fallen and broken his hip; a forty-eight-year-old man with abdominal pain and rectal bleeding.

At midnight, a woman arrived complaining of squeezing chest pain; at 2 a.m., a sixty-two-year-old man with known cancer arrived with a high fever; at two thirty, a schoolteacher who had had abdominal surgery two months before was admitted with symptoms of small-bowel obstruction.

The last resident got to bed shortly before 5 a.m., lying fully dressed on a stretcher in one of the treatment rooms. On his door was tacked a sheet of paper which said "Wake me at 6:30."

✠

"However great the kindness and the efficiency," wrote George Orwell, "in every hospital death there will be some cruel, squalid detail, something perhaps too small

to be told but leaving terribly painful memories behind, arising out of the haste, the crowding, the impersonality of a place where every day people are dying
among strangers."

That is a reasonable description of Ralph Orlando's
death, and the unfortunate way his family learned of it.
Yet one cannot imagine those events taking place anywhere in the hospital except in the emergency ward.
The EW is the place where the haste, the crowding, and
the impersonality are seen in their most exaggerated
form. And in many ways, the EW is the place where
one can see most clearly the work that the hospital per-
forms, in all its positive and negative aspects; the EW
is a kind of microcosm for the hospital as a whole. Its
growth in recent years has been phenomenal. Its patient
load has been increasing steadily at a rate of 10 per cent
per year for nearly a decade. It now treats more than
65,000 patients a year. Half of all hospital admissions
come through the emergency ward, and many aspects of
hospital life are now arranged around that fact: for example, elective admissions in medicine and surgery may
have to wait as long as twelve weeks for a free bed,
because emergency cases receive priority. If an elective
patient has, for example, surgically treatable cancer, the
delay may be difficult for everyone to accept.

Yet the trend is clear. The hospital is oriented toward
curative treatment of established disease at an advanced
or critical stage. Increasingly, the hospital population
tends to consist of patients with more and more acute

illnesses, until even cancer must accept a somewhat secondary position. And there is no indication that the hospital has fallen into this role passively; on the contrary, this appears to be the logical outcome of many aspects of its evolution.

✠

Massachusetts General Hospital now consists of twenty-one buildings along the banks of the Charles River. Included within this complex are the first structure, the Bulfinch Building, and the most recent, the Gray Building and Jackson Towers, still under construction. All together, the hospital has more than 1,000 beds, and is one of the largest hospitals in the United States.

Invisible is a complex of equal size, consisting of all the buildings that have been erected and then torn down during the last hundred and forty-six years—the isolation wards, the Building for Offensive Diseases, the laboratories and operating rooms that have come and gone as the demands of medical practice and the patterns of disease have shifted.

The hospital is now so large and so busy that it is difficult to grasp the magnitude of its activity. In 1967, it admitted 27,000 patients, performed 16,000 operations, treated 62,000 people in its emergency ward, examined 115,000 patients by X ray, saw 226,000 clinic patients, and dispensed 176,000 prescriptions from its pharmacy. These figures are so large as to be almost meaningless.

A better way to look at the job the hospital does is to view it on the basis of a twenty-four-hour day, three hundred sixty-five days a year. On that basis, the hospital sees a new patient in the emergency ward every eight minutes. X rays are taken on a patient every five minutes. A new patient is admitted every twenty minutes. And a new operation is begun every thirty minutes.

The hospital's operating budget is some $35 million yearly. It has grown so expensive, in fact, that the initial sum of $140,000 that was used to build the hospital in 1821 now could not support its operation for a day and a half.

The growth in patient care has been equalled by a growth in teaching activity. From a handful of medical students following a senior man from patient to patient in 1821, the hospital's student population has grown to more than 800, including 250 medical students, 304 interns and residents, and 339 nursing students.

Added to these two traditional concerns—patient care and teaching—has been a third purpose: research. Here the growth has been both recent and phenomenal. As late as 1935, the MGH research budget was $44,000. By 1967, it was $10.5 million, with another $1.3 million for indirect costs of research. The research activities have transformed the very nature of the institution, making it, in combination with the medical school, a complete system for medical advance. Discoveries are made here; they are applied to patients; and new generations of physicians are trained in the new techniques.

It is this orientation toward innovation, and this commitment to scientific advancement, that the teaching hospital has contributed to the long history of hospitals. In other areas of its development, such as the emphasis on emergency care, the teaching hospital shares a trend evident among all hospitals everywhere, though it displays the trend in a more pronounced form.

✠

The evolution of the hospital has been going on for more than two thousand years, beginning with the first system of hospitals about which much is known, the *aesculapia* of Greece. These first appeared around 350 B.C., taking the form of temples to Aesculapius, a deified physician who had lived nearly a thousand years earlier. (Homer insists that Aesculapius was a mortal, despite the fact that he was a pupil of the centaur Chiron.) The legendary fate of Aesculapius is ironic, for it represents the first statement that good medical care could lead to population problems. According to legend, Aesculapius was so successful as a healer that Hades became depopulated; Pluto complained to Zeus, who eliminated Aesculapius with a thunderbolt. The Aesculapian temples were not so much hospitals as religious institutions where patients came on pilgrimages, hoping to be cured by a

visitation of the gods; the medical historian Henry Sigerist suggests Lourdes as the closest modern parallel.

Predictably, the most common cures were of people
suffering from what would now be called hysterical or
psychosomatic illness—headache, insomnia, indigestion,
blindness caused by emotional trauma, and so on.

The hospital in a more modern sense began in late
Roman times, and coincided with the spread of Christianity across Europe. The word "hospital" is derived
from the Latin *hospes*, meaning host or guest; the same
root has given us "hotel" and "hostel." Indeed, the
first hospitals were little different from hotels and hos-
tels. Essentially they were places where the sick could
rest and be fed until they recuperated or died. All
hospitals were run by the Church, and most were associated with monasteries. Medicine was practiced by
monks and priests.

In theory, Sigerist notes, "Christianity gave the sick
man a position in society that he had never had before, a
preferential position. When Christianity became the official religion of the Roman Empire, society as such became responsible for the care of the sick."

But in practice, this preferential position had its drawbacks. Conditions in the medieval hospitals varied
widely. Certain of them, well financed and well managed, were famous for their humane treatment and their
cheerful, spacious surroundings. But most were essentially custodial institutions to keep troublesome and
infectious people off the streets. In these places, crowd-

24

ing, filth, and high mortality among both patients and attendants were the rule.

All this soon led to the notion that one avoided a hospital if at all possible. Wealthier—and more worldly —patients were treated in their homes by apothecaries and barber surgeons; only the traveler, the very poor, and the hopelessly ill found their way into the hospitals, and for these people it was indeed "an antechamber to the tomb."

The Renaissance and Reformation loosened the Church's strong hold on both the hospital and the conduct of medical practice. New medical schools sprang up at Salerno, Bologna, Montpellier, and Oxford; in England, Henry VIII dissolved the monastery-hospital system altogether, and a network of private, nonprofit, voluntary hospitals was started to take its place.

A medical school was associated with St. Bartholomew's in 1622; it has thus been a teaching hospital for nearly three hundred and fifty years. Among its eminent surgeons and physicians have been William Harvey, the discoverer of the circulation of the blood; Percival Pott, who first described Pott's disease, tuberculosis of the spine; the brilliant and inventive surgeon John Abernethy, and Sir James Paget, the man who described Paget's disease.

During the seventeenth century, urban London was growing enormously, yet there were only two hospitals —St. Bartholomew's and St. Thomas's. The demands made upon these two institutions gradually resulted in

25

an important change in function. Instead of caring for all patients, they shifted their emphasis to patients who could be cured, leaving the incurables to asylums and prisons. In 1700, St. Thomas's orders stated flatly: "No incurables are to be received"—a harsh order, but one with the encouraging implication that medicine was beginning to divide its clientele into those who could be helped, and those who could not. The situation was made more humane a few years later when a wealthy merchant, Sir Thomas Guy, financed one of the first private, voluntary hospitals to care for all patients, curable or not.

By now the hospital was becoming demonstrably more modern in purpose, but it remained a place to be feared and shunned. George Orwell notes that "if you look at almost any literature before the latter part of the nineteenth century, you find that a hospital is popularly regarded as much the same thing as a prison, and an old-fashioned, dungeon-like prison at that. A hospital is a place of filth, torture, and death, a sort of antechamber to the tomb. No one who was not more or less destitute would have thought of going into such a place for treatment."

Under the circumstances, it is not surprising that the first American colonists were in no hurry to build hospitals.

✠

Although there was only one physician among the original passengers on the *Mayflower*, generally speaking the early immigrants to Massachusetts were remarkably well educated. According to one estimate, in 1640 there was an Oxford or Cambridge graduate for every two hundred and fifty colonists. This may have been the reason why Massachusetts had the first college (Harvard, 1636), the first printing press (in Cambridge, 1639), and the first newspaper in the Colonies (Boston, 1704). Massachusetts also contributed the first medical article written and published in the New World—"A Brief Rule to Guide the Common People of New England how to order themselves and theirs in the Small-Pocks, or Measels." It was written by Thomas Thacher, the first minister of the Old South Church. (Not all the energies of the colonists were directed toward intellectual pursuits, however, for Massachusetts also contributed the first epidemic of syphilis in the New World, in Boston, 1646.)

Nevertheless, Boston had no general hospital for two hundred years after the landing of the Pilgrims. During this time the city had been growing rapidly—from a population of 4,500 in 1680, to 11,000 in 1720, and finally to 32,896 in 1810. By now it was clear that an almshouse was inadequate for the population, a conclusion reached some years earlier in the larger cities of Philadelphia and New York.

Thus the Reverend John Bartlett, chaplain of the overcrowded almshouse, wrote a letter in 1811 to "fifteen or twenty-five of the wealthiest and most respected citizens of Boston," urging support of a general hospital. Shortly before, two professors of the newly formed Harvard Medical School had written a similar letter. Their emphasis was slightly different, for the medical school needed a hospital for clinical teaching, and every attempt to use the existing almshouse or to build a new hospital had been blocked by the local medical society, whose members feared the encroachment of the school on the conduct of medical practice.

Through these letters run a number of recurrent themes: that a hospital is indispensable for training young doctors; that existing facilities are inadequate; that the obligations of Christian charity demand support of a hospital; and that Boston has fallen behind Philadelphia and New York.

The appeal, on many levels, was certainly successful. When fund-raising began in 1816 (it was delayed by the War of 1812), $78,802 was collected in the first three days, the donations eventually exceeded $140,000.

The State was involved to the following extent: it granted a charter to incorporate the Massachusetts General Hospital; it contributed some real estate along the banks of the Charles River; it contributed granite for construction of the building; and it supplied convict labor to build it.

The designer of the building was Charles Bulfinch, Jr., a leading architect and son of a prominent physician. With its dome, the building was an architectural

28

marvel of its time, and was considered the most beautiful structure in Boston for many years afterward. Organizationally, too, it was quite advanced; it was patterned upon the English urban teaching hospital as exemplified by Guy's Hospital in London.

The new institution was not, however, immediately popular with Boston citizenry. The first patient appeared on September 3, 1821, but no other applied until September 20, and the hospital never ran at full census until after 1850, when massive emigration from Ireland increased the city population fourfold.

This early reluctance to use the newly founded institution is frequently attributed to experiences with earlier hospitals, such as the military hospitals of the Revolution (which Benjamin Rush said "robbed the United States of more citizens than the sword"), the pesthouses, and the almshouses. But in fact it is perfectly understandable if one considers the state of medical science when the hospital first opened its doors.

In 1821, the concept that cleanliness could prevent infection was unknown. There was little systematic attempt to keep the hospital clean; physicians went directly from the autopsy room to the bedside without washing their hands, and surgeons operated in whatever old street clothes were considered too shabby for other purposes.

In 1821, the stethoscope was a newfangled French gadget, invented four years before by Laënnec. (It was a hollow tube, designed to break into two pieces so it could be carried inside a physician's top hat.) The syringe for injection was a novelty; the clinical thermometer would not be introduced for another forty years; and X-ray diagnosis was nearly a century off.

In 1821, the average physician's list of drugs contained many substances of doubtful value, including live worms, oil of ants, snakeskins, strychnine, bile, and human perspiration. No so long previously, Governor John Winthrop had accepted powdered unicorn horn as a valuable addition to his pharmacopoeia. And if all this seems an exaggeration, it is worth remembering that as late as 1910 some doctors at the hospital still regarded strychnine as good treatment for pneumonia.

In 1821, there was no anesthesia, and consequently few operations. The post-operative infection rate was nearly 100 per cent. Surgical mortality was close to 80 per cent. In the first full year of service, the hospital treated 115 patients. Although records from that time are lost, the mortality for the hospital as a whole in its early years was a fairly constant 10 per cent.

Clearly, the hospital has undergone an astonishing growth in size and complexity since those days. That growth generally goes unquestioned; it is a peculiarity of the American mentality that the growth of almost anything is applauded. (Consider the mindless jubilation that accompanied the growth of our population to two hundred million.) One may ask whether there are any drawbacks to the size of today's MGH, and to its current emphasis on acute, curative medicine. The question is difficult to answer.

First there is size. For both patient and physician, the sheer size of the hospital can create problems. The patient may find it cold, enormous, impersonal; the doctor whose patients or consultations are widely scattered may find himself walking as much as a quarter of a mile from bed to bed. The intimate, supportive atmosphere that is possible in a smaller hospital cannot be achieved to the same extent here.

On the other hand, a large patient population permits active research on a range of less common diseases; and the hospital serves a genuine function as a place of expert management in such illnesses. Similarly, highly technical procedures, requiring trained personnel and expensive machinery, can be supported in a large hospital, and these procedures can be carried out with a high degree of expertise. Patients who require open-heart surgery or sophisticated radiotherapy find the expensive equipment for such procedures here—and, equally important, staff that carries out such procedures daily.

As for the emphasis on curative measures directed toward established organic illness, two points can be made. First, the hospital's ability to continue to care for the patient once he has left the hospital is not as good as anyone would like. The MGH founded the first social-service department in America, in 1905, to look after such follow-up care in areas not strictly medical. These departments are now standard in most large hospitals.

Similarly, the out-patient clinics are designed to provide continuity of medical care to ambulatory patients. But many patients are "lost to follow-up," to use the hospital's expression; they don't answer the social worker's calls, or they don't keep their clinic appointment. Nor can they be wholly faulted in this regard, for the hospital's out-patient services are, in general, quite time-consuming for the person who wants to use them. Not only does the patient spend hours in the clinic itself, but he must take the time to travel to and from the hospital on each visit.

Second, by definition the hospital has not done much in the area of preventive medicine. No hospital ever has. Since the *aesculapia*, hospitals have defined themselves as passive institutions, taking whoever comes to them but seeking no one out. There are some peculiar side-lights to this. For example, a high percentage of patients in the acute psychiatric service give a family history of severe psychiatric disturbance. In the case of the young girl who had tried to kill her child, her father was an alcoholic; her mother and younger brother had committed suicide; her twenty-year-old husband, a shoe salesman, had recently been admitted to a state hospital for an acute psychotic break.

It is possible to think of psychiatric illness as almost infectious, in the sense that these disorders are so frequently self-perpetuating. One is tempted to reflect that true infectious disease is best treated in the community, using direct preventive and therapeutic measures; indeed, the conquest of infectious disease—one of the triumphs of medicine in this century—is something for which the hospital, as an institution, can take no credit at all.

In the same way, it is in the hospital's approach to mental illness that its limitations as a curative institution, treating already established disease, are today most striking. If major inroads are to be made, they will not come from the hospital system as it is presently structured, any more than the old specialized hospitals for tuberculosis, leprosy, and smallpox had any real impact on the decline of those diseases.

Some of the ways the hospital is restructuring itself to meet these limitations will be discussed later. But the hospital is also revising its internal workings, and that is the subject of the next chapter.

JOHN O'CONNOR

Until his admission, John O'Connor, a fifty-year-old railroad dispatcher from Charlestown, was in perfect health. He had never been sick a day in his life.

On the morning of his admission, he awoke early, complaining of vague abdominal pain. He vomited once, bringing up clear material, and had some diarrhea. He went to see his family doctor, who said that he had no fever and his white cell count was normal. He told Mr. O'Connor that it was probably gastroenteritis, and advised him to rest and take paregoric to settle his stomach.

In the afternoon, Mr. O'Connor began to feel warm. He then had two shaking chills. His wife suggested he call his doctor once again, but when Mr. O'Connor went to the phone, he collapsed. At 5 p.m. his wife brought him to the MGH emergency ward, where he was noted to have a temperature of 108° F. and a white count of 37,000 (normal count: 5,000–10,000).

The patient was wildly delirious; it required ten people to hold him down as he thrashed about. He spoke only nonsense words and groans, and did not respond to his name. While in the emergency ward he had massive diarrhea consisting of several quarts of watery fluid.

The patient was seen by the medical resident, John Minna, who instituted immediate therapy consisting of aspirin, alcohol rubs, fans and a refrigerating blanket to bring down his fever, which rapidly fell to 100°. He was in shock with an initial blood pressure of 70/30 and a central venous pressure of zero. Over the next three hours he received three quarts of plasma and two quarts of salt water intravenously, to replace fluids lost from sweating and diarrhea. He was also severely acidotic, so he was given twelve ampoules of intravenous sodium bicarbonate as well as potassium chloride to correct an electrolyte balance.

The patient could not give a history. His wife, upon questioning, denied any history of malaria, distant travel, food exposure, infectious disease, headache, neck stiffness, cough, sputum, sore throat, swollen glands, arthritis, muscle aches, seizures, skin infection, drug ingestion or past suicide attempts.

His past history, according to the wife, was unremarkable. He had never been ill or hospitalized. His mother died at age fifty-five of leukemia; his father at age fifty-nine, of pneumonia. The patient had no known allergies, and did not smoke or drink.

Physical examination was normal except for a slightly distended abdomen and a questionably enlarged liver, which could be felt below the rib cage. Neurological examination was normal except for the patient's stuporous, unresponsive mental state.

The patient was cultured "stem to stern," meaning that samples of blood, urine, stool, sputum, and spinal fluid were sent for bacteriological analysis. He was also given heavy doses of antibiotics, including a gram of chloramphenicol, a gram of oxacillin, two million units of penicillin; later in the evening, kanamycin and colistin were added to the list.

X rays of the chest and abdomen were normal. Electrocardiogram was normal. Hematocrit was normal. The white count was elevated at 37,000 with a preponderance of polymorphonuclear leukocytes, the cells which increase in bacterial infections. Examination of the urine showed a few white cells. Platelet count and prothrombin time were normal. Measurements of blood sugar, serum amylase, serum acetone, bilirubin, blood urea nitrogen were normal. Lumbar puncture was normal.

An intravenous pyelogram (an X ray of the kidneys to check their function while they excrete an opaque dye) showed that the left kidney was normal, but the right kidney responded sluggishly. The excretory tubing on the right side seemed dilated. A diagnosis of partial obstruction of the right kidney system was suggested.

Because the abdomen was distended, six abdominal taps were performed in different areas by the surgical residents, Drs. Robert Corry and Jay Kaufman, in an attempt to obtain fluid from the abdominal cavity. None was obtained.

Dr. Minna's diagnosis was septicemia, or generalized infection of the bloodstream, from an unknown source. As possibilities he listed the urinary tract, the gastrointestinal tract, the gall bladder, or the lining of the heart. He felt that there was no good evidence for a central nervous system cause for the fever, and no good history of drug ingestion or thyroid problems to account for the fever.

This was essentially the conclusion of the neurological consultants who saw the patient later in the evening. They felt that Mr. O'Connor had suffered a primary infectious process with sudden outpouring of bacteria into the blood, and consequent fever and prostration. They felt the infection was somewhere in the urinary or gastrointestinal system, or perhaps even in a small area of the lungs. In their opinion, meningitis, encephalitis, subarachnoid hemorrhage, or other central nervous problems were unlikely.

A formal surgical consult, also later in the evening, reported that in the absence of muscle spasm or guarding of the abdomen, and in the presence of six negative taps, an acute abdominal crisis was unlikely.

Genito-urinary consultants examined the patient that same evening and reviewed his kidney X rays. They felt that there was a probable partial obstruction of the right kidney, but they could not determine whether this was a recent or a slowly developing change. They found no evidence of infection of the prostate gland to explain the fever.

Mr. O'Connor was placed on the Danger List and transferred to the intensive-care unit of the Bulfinch Building. At the end of his first twelve hours in the hospital, his fever had been reduced, but was still unexplained.

✠

Before continuing with Mr. O'Connor's hospital course, it is worth pausing a moment to consider the patient's initial symptoms, and initial therapy.

Mr. O'Connor presented with high fever and shock. Classically, the fever of unknown origin is a pediatric problem, and classically it is a problem for the same reasons it was a problem with Mr. O'Connor—the patient cannot tell you how he feels or what hurts. However, a high fever in a child is less worrisome than it is in an adult, for children have a much greater tolerance for fever. In adults, prolonged high fever is more likely to result in permanent brain damage and death.

The most common cause of fever for anyone, child or adult, is infection; the most common cause of fever of unknown origin is also infection. There are some unusual causes occasionally seen, such as malignancies, bleeding in the brain, drug ingestion, and outpouring of thyroid hormone, but, for the most part, unexplained fevers are produced by unidentified infections.

It is now known that one can harbor an infection in a secluded part of the body, and the body will make very little response to it; however, if the infection spreads into the bloodstream, there may be a "shower" of bacteria, and a subsequent rise in temperature. The shower is usually brief, lasting minutes or hours, and often ends before the temperature rises. This make diagnosis difficult—if one wants to catch bacteria in the blood, one must draw a sample *before* the temperature spike, and not during it or after it.

It was thought that Mr. O'Connor was suffering from precisely this sort of situation: a sequestered infection producing episodic bursts of bacteria into the blood, with episodic fever. However, his fever was threateningly high. And thus a classic conflict in therapy as old as Hippocrates.

"For extreme diseases, extreme remedies," Hippocrates wrote. But he also said: "For grave diseases, the most exact therapy is best." But, obviously, an exact therapy depends upon a precise diagnosis, and here lies the conflict.

What is a diagnosis? The question is not as simpleminded as it first appears, for the notion of what constitutes an acceptable diagnosis has radically changed through the years.

A diagnosis is drawn up on the basis of two kinds of knowledge: the physician's concept of disease processes, and his available therapies. Ideally, a diagnosis contains some sense of etiology—the cause of the disease—but for most of medical history etiology was either ignored or wrongly ascribed (as in "fever from excess of black bile").

In a modern sense, precise diagnosis is required because precise therapies are available. Yet the need for precise diagnosis is older; in Hippocratic time, this need was based on a prognostic, not a therapeutic, concern. Physicians were unskilled at curing disease and therefore served mostly to predict the course of an illness which they could not influence. Robert Platt notes that "until quite recently . . . it did not matter whether your diagnosis was right or wrong. . . . Prognosis mattered rather more, especially to the doctor's reputation."

Hippocrates was deeply concerned with the prestige of the physician as related to prognostic acumen; much Hippocratic writing shows this preoccupation with prognosis: "Sleep following upon delirium is a good sign." "Those who swoon frequently without apparent cause are liable to die suddenly." "Labored sleep in any disease is a bad sign." "Spasm supervening upon a wound is dangerous." "Hardening of the liver in jaundice is bad." "If a convalescent eats heartily, yet does not take on flesh, it is a bad sign."

43

These observations are still valid today. But we demand something further from diagnosis, as the range of therapies has increased. If a person swoons, for example, it is important to know whether he has aortic stenosis—and is likely to die suddenly—or whether he is hysterical, or diabetic, or has some other reason for fainting. In short, we want more precise diagnoses because we have more precise therapies.

Throughout medical history, physicians have felt that they had precise, specific remedies, but few of these are still acceptable. As medical writer Berton Roueché notes, only three eighteenth-century drugs are still acceptable today: quinine for malaria, colchicine for gout, and foxglove (digitalis) for heart failure. All the other "specifics," as well as what Holmes termed the "peremptory drastics," have disappeared.

Even as recently as 1910, L. J. Henderson commented that "if the average patient visited the average physician, he would have a fifty-fifty chance of benefiting from the encounter." Much has happened since then—in fact, nearly every diagnostic test and therapeutic procedure performed on Mr. O'Connor during those first twelve hours has been developed since 1910. For clinically, diagnosis and therapy go hand in hand; increasing sophistication in either one demands increased sophistication in the other.

The proliferation of tests and techniques in this century is staggering. Consider the following list of tests per-

44

formed on Mr. O'Connor, and the dates those tests were
first described in clinically practical terms:

  X ray: chest and abdomen (1905–15)
  White cell count (about 1895)
  Serum acetone (1928)
  Amylase (1948)
  Calcium (1931)
  Phosphorus (1925)
  SGOT (1955)
  LDH(1956)
  CPK (1961)
  Aldolase (1949)
  Lipase (1934)
  CSF protein (1931)
  CSF sugar (1932)
  Blood sugar (1932)
  Bilirubin (1937)
  Serum albumin/globulin (1923–38)
  Electrolytes (1941–6)
  Electrocardiogram (about 1915)
  Prothrombin time (1940)
  Blood pH (1924–57)
  Blood gases (1957)
  Protein-bound iodine (1948)
  Alkaline phosphatase (1933)
  Watson-Schwartz (1941)
  Creatinine (1933)
  Uric acid (1933)

If one were to graph these tests, and others commonly
used, against the total time course of medical history,

one would see a flat line for more than two thousand years, followed by a slight rise beginning about 1850, and then an ever-sharper rise to the present time.

That is the meaning of technological innovation. It has struck medicine like a thunderbolt: far more advances have occurred in medicine in the last hundred years than occurred in the previous two thousand. There is no mystery why this should be so. Most research scientists in history are alive today; therefore most of the discoveries in history are being made today. But the consequences of this vast outpouring of information and technology have yet to be grasped. Major questions are raised in such widely diverse subjects as medical education and euthanasia.

What makes the case of Mr. O'Connor so interesting is the way it illustrates the vast web of technological advances that make diagnostic techniques and treatment today so radically different from what they were only thirty years ago.

✠

Presumably, Mr. O'Connor had an infection. The treatment of infectious disease is considered one of the triumphs of modern medicine, crowned by the introduction of antibiotics. But as the bacteriologist René Dubos has pointed out, "The decrease in mortality caused by infection began nearly a century ago and has

46

continued ever since at a fairly constant rate irrespective of the use of any specific therapy." He says, further, that "these triumphs of modern chemotherapy have transformed the practice of medicine and are changing the very pattern of disease in the western world, but there is no reason to believe that they spell the *conquest* of microbial diseases."

In this light, consider Mr. O'Connor's antibiotic "cocktail," given shortly after admission. It was later the subject of some heated discussion when, during the first two or three days, he failed to improve.

The use of antibiotics is more sophisticated now than it was twenty years ago, corresponding to a better appraisal of the benefits and limitations of the drugs. Generally speaking, the antibiotic cocktail, a mixture of drugs given before one has diagnosed the nature of the infection, is frowned upon.

The arguments against it are simple enough. For Mr. O'Connor, the mixture of antibiotics might not eliminate the primary site of infection—but it would certainly kill all free bacteria in the blood, thus making identification of the organisms impossible. Without identification, one cannot treat specifically, by matching the organism with the single most effective antibiotic. Further, the inability to identify the organism deprives doctors of an important clue to the location of the infection, since different organisms are more likely to infect different parts of the body.

47

The arguments in favor of the cocktail are equally simple: that Mr. O'Connor's fever was, in itself, dangerous and constituted a medical emergency. The first duty of the EW residents, as they saw it, was to lower that fever by every possible means, even if this hampered further diagnostic efforts. As one resident said, "He could have died while we waited for the cultures to grow out."

It all comes back to Hippocrates: Does one treat with a grave remedy, or a specific one? The MGH chose a grave remedy, a strong antibiotic cocktail. The residents did so with the full knowledge that it might impair further work.

Let us now see what happened to Mr. O'Connor.

✠

DAY 1

Mr. O'Connor survived the night. The following morning his blood pressure was normal and his temperature was 99°, but he remained severely agitated and unresponsive. He was sedated with morphine, continued on intravenous fluids and electrolyte supplements. The oxygenation of his blood had been poor from the start and he was continued on oxygen by face mask.

At eight in the morning the genito-urinary consult saw him and felt that he had peritonitis of the right abdomen, or infection of the sac-like membrane which sur-

48

rounds the abdominal contents. Evidence included tenderness and muscle spasm on the right side, and tenderness when his liver was tapped. Bowel sounds were decreased, suggestive of intra-abdominal infection. There was tenderness to rectal examination, also suggestive of such infection.

At nine, Dr. Minna examined the patient again and agreed that the tenderness was impressive, particularly after a heavy dose of morphine. An X-ray study of the gall bladder was planned. At eleven, he was seen by the surgeons who agreed that gall-bladder infection was possible, even though bilirubin and amylase tests were normal. They advised waiting on surgery, however.

At noon, the gastrointestinal consult reviewed the barium enema, which was normal. They concluded that "we remain in the dark regarding diagnosis but would agree that bacterial sepsis secondary to a right abdominal lesion is the best bet." They suggested, however, that perforated small bowel, duodenal lesion, pancreatitis, and a number of other possibilities remained, and advised an upper GI series of X rays.

At approximately the same time, the attending physician on the wards, Dr. Kurt Bloch, noted that Mr. O'Connor presented "a very puzzling problem," with some findings suggestive of right-upper-abdomen pathology, but no clear indication of what it might be.

Later in the day the surgeons again saw Mr. O'Connor, but disagreed with earlier interpretations. They felt his abdomen had no peritoneal signs, and no localizing signs.

At eight in the evening, the neuromedical consult again evaluated Mr. O'Connor, and concluded that his condition still gave no hint of central nervous system disease. They felt that findings pointed to an abdominal problem.

That same evening, more abnormal laboratory values came back from the labs. They had been taken the day of admission, and included an elevated uric acid level of 17.1 and an elevated alkaline phosphatase level of 37.6. The alkaline phosphatase test was repeated, and was found to be still higher, at 61.0. Two other enzymes were also slightly high: the serum glutamic oxalocetic transaminase, or SGOT, was 123, and the lactic dehydrogenase, or LDH, was 540. Blood samples were immediately drawn for repeat determinations.

These two enzymes, SGOT and LDH, are measured as indexes of cell destruction. Cells normally contain them; if the cells die, they rupture and release their enzymes to the bloodstream. A rise in enzyme levels is thought to correspond moderately well with the degree of cellular damage, particularly when followed over several days. However, these enzymes are found in many kinds of cells, and thus an enzyme rise does not pinpoint precisely the area of destruction. For example, heart, skeletal muscle, brain, liver, and kidneys all contain SGOT; damage to any of them will produce an SGOT rise. In recent years, there has been a search for enzymes specific to certain tissues. Creatinine phosphokinase, or CPK, is usually considered more specific for heart damage.

DAY 2

At 3:30 a.m., Michael Soper, a medical resident, got back the new set of enzyme values. Everything was further increased: SGOT was now 640, LDH 1250, and CPK very high, at 320. He wrote: "I've never seen a CPK this high and don't know where it is coming from. Doubt it is solely of cardiac origin. Electrocardiogram tonight is unchanged."

At 7 a.m., on morning rounds, Mr. O'Connor's abdomen was again without localizing signs pointing to disease on the right side. All cultures were back from the labs; all were negative. It was decided to continue only penicillin and chloramphenicol, and discontinue all other antibiotics.

Later in the morning, the patient was seen by the infectious-disease consult, which concluded that the agitation and unresponsiveness were almost certainly secondary to gastrointestinal disorders and metabolic problems. The elevated enzymes could be the consequence of insufficient oxygen and shock, present at admission. However, they noted that the elevated alkaline phosphatase and elevated uric acid were unexplained.

51

They suggested the possibility, previously unconsidered, of staphylococcal food poisoning.

Since no information could be obtained directly from the patient, his wife was closely requestioned about symptoms of thyroid disease, or long-standing diarrhea or other GI problems. The paregoric that the patient had taken on the day of admission was brought into the hospital and checked; it was, indeed, paregoric.

During this period the patient was examined by Dr. Alexander Leaf, the chief of medicine, and Dr. Daniel Federman, the assistant chief, as well as by a large number of other physicians, in an informal brainstorming session. Every conceivable diagnosis, including mushroom poisoning and cholera, was considered at this time.

The patient's condition remained unchanged.

DAY 3

Continued problems with oxygenating the patient's bloodstream produced a consultation by the respiratory unit, which advised drying the lungs as much as possible, naso-tracheal suctioning, encouraging coughing, and close monitoring by arterial blood gases. The patient improved somewhat during the day, becoming less wild. That evening, for the first time, he responded to his name.

DAY 4

The patient was more alert. He was seen again by the surgeons, who noted his abdomen was still soft, without any indications for surgery. His dose of Valium, to contain his agitation, was reduced.

DAY 5

He was seen in the morning by the neurological consults, who felt that he was "still quite obtunded," confused and disoriented. Nonetheless his progress since admission was striking. He could answer questions. When asked where he was, he said, "The hospital," though he could not specify which one. When asked his name, he said, "John." He could state his age. He was taken off Valium entirely. His temperature continued to fluctuate in the range of 99°–101° F. Dr. Minna wrote: "He is better in all ways."

DAY 6

Lab values, back from the day before, continued to climb. CPK had now gone to 2900, the highest in the history of the hospital. There was still no explanation for these enzyme changes. The patient continued to improve in alertness and responsiveness, though his mental function was far from satisfactory. In answer to questions, he said that one plus one was "one," and two plus two was "five."

DAY 7

He was able to carry out verbal commands such as "Squeeze my hand" and "Open your eyes." However,

53

for the most part he lay in bed with his eyes closed; he initiated little spontaneous activity, and never spoke except in reply to questions.

DAY 8

His Foley catheter was removed. He was able to urinate in the normal manner. He was more active mentally, and remembered his last name, for the first time.

DAY 9

Blood cultures now revealed growth of a gramnegative bacillus, identified as *Bactroides*, probably of bowel origin. The patient was sufficiently improved that he could be questioned about toxins, drugs, mushrooms, work exposure, and possible ingestions of heavy metals; there was no evidence for any of these. He was seen again by surgeons, who concluded that his abdomen was soft, with normal bowel sounds.

DAY 10

He was seen by the neurological consults, who observed mild proximal muscle weakness and suggested study of the electrical activity of the muscles, by electromyography. He was also noted to have mushy swelling of his extremities.

DAY 11

The patient's mental condition continued to improve. A repeat kidney X ray was read as normal.

54

DAY 12

There was continued improvement. Enzymes had dropped to near-normal levels. He had no fever.

DAY 13

Barium enema was repeated, looking for diverticulitis or other sources of infection. None was seen.

DAY 14

Electromyography was normal. It was decided to discontinue his chloramphenicol antibiotic and see if he remained without fever.

DAY 15

Chloramphenicol was stopped. The patient did well, taking liquids by mouth.

DAY 16

On his second day off antibiotics, his temperature fluctuated in the range of 100°–101° F.

DAY 17

The patient had an upper gastrointestinal series of X rays, which were normal. On his third day off antibiotics, the temperature began to spike again, to 102°. Tenderness and guarding of the right-upper abdomen reappeared.

DAY 18

The surgeons concluded that the patient had cholecystitis, or infection of the gall bladder, which had probably begun initially as cholangitis, infection of the bile system. They also wondered, however, whether he might have a liver abscess. The patient was put back on antibiotics.

DAY 19

Mr. O'Connor was transferred from the medical service to the surgical service as a pre-operative candidate for exploratory abdominal surgery. His mental state continued to clear slowly.

DAY 20

The neurological consult saw him and agreed his mental status was improving. The surgeons, moreover, found that his abdominal tenderness had disappeared with the antibiotics. X rays of the gall bladder showed no filling of the bladder sac, but the films were of poor quality. Radioactive scans of the liver and spleen were negative.

DAY 21

The scheduled operation was canceled in order to allow time for further pre-operative studies. A repeated gall bladder X ray definitely showed no filling, although this time the films were of good quality. A celiac angiogram was scheduled.

DAY 22 and DAY 23

The weekend. Specialized procedures such as celiac angiography could not be done, and further work on the patient was postponed until Monday.

DAY 24

Celiac angiography was performed. Under local anesthetic, a thin, flexible catheter was passed up the femoral artery in the leg, to the aorta, and finally to the celiac axis, a network of arteries coming off the aorta to supply blood to all the upper-abdominal organs. A dye opaque to X rays was injected, and the vessels studied. No space-occupying lesion (tumor) was found and the vessels were normal in appearance. The patient made a good recovery from the procedure.

DAY 25

The abdomen was soft and non-tender. The patient felt well. He was still on chloramphenicol. Enzymes were, by now, fully normal.

DAY 26

The patient had no fever and felt well. The surgical staff decided to stop antibiotics and see if fever and symptoms recurred.

DAY 27

He was taken off antibiotics. Temperature and

57

white cell count remained normal. The patient himself was in good spirits.

DAY 28

There was no demonstrable worsening of the patient's condition on his second day off antibiotics. His wife expressed the opinion that his mental state was entirely normal once more.

DAY 29

His condition remained stable on the third day. He said he felt well. He had no fever and no elevation in white count.

DAY 30

His condition was still good; his abdomen was soft without tenderness. He said he felt well. It was now clear that he was not an operative candidate. Plans were made for his discharge the following day.

DAY 31

Discharged. His discharge diagnosis was fever of unknown origin with bacteroides septicemia. The opinion of the house staff remained that this patient had probably had a bile-collecting-system infection.

Five days after discharge, he was seen in the surgical clinic by Dr. Jack Monchik, who scheduled another set of gall bladder X rays for the future, and noted that if the patient had further trouble with infection, it would probably be necessary to remove the gall bladder. For the moment, however, the patient was fully well.

❋

"To do nothing," said Hippocrates, "is sometimes a good remedy."

On the surface, Mr. O'Connor's hospital course seems proof of this ancient dictum of "watchful waiting." But this is not really so: had Mr. O'Connor received no treatment, he would almost certainly have died within twenty-four hours. He received vital symptomatic therapy (lowering his fever) as well as acute support of vital functions (assisted respiration). He was closely monitored by teams of physicians who were prepared to intercede in his behalf, supplying more assistance should his body require it.

He also received a vigorous diagnostic work-up, which did not produce as much information as one might like. His therapy was successful, but no physician at the hospital could claim, at discharge, that they really knew what was going on in his case. A diagnosis of cholangitis and cholecystitis was likely, but never demonstrated.

His hospital bill for a month of care was $6,172.55. This is just a few dollars less than Mr. O'Connor's annual salary. But he did not have to worry about it; unlike most patient with some form of health insurance,

Mr. O'Connor had coverage that was essentially complete. His personal bill amounted to $357.00.

In this, as in many other things, Mr. O'Connor was a very lucky man.

One portion of Mr. O'Connor's 17-foot-long bill:

POSTING DATE		CHARGE DESCRIPTION		TOTAL CHARGE	INSURANCE COVERAGE	CHARGE TO PATIENT
MONTH	DAY					
06	05	CHEM-LAB	0548209 F	4.00	4.00	
06	05	CHEM-LAB	0548243 F	2.50	2.50	
06	05	CHEM-LAB	0548290 F	6.00	6.00	
06	05	CHEM-LAB	0548294 F	2.00	2.00	
06	05	CHEM-LAB	0548359 F	2.00	2.00	
06	05	CHEM-LAB	0548361 F	5.00	5.00	
06	05	CHEM-LAB	0548367 F	2.50	2.50	
06	05	CHEM-LAB	0548407 F	2.00	2.00	
06	05	CHEM-LAB	0548431 F	2.00	2.00	
06	05	CHEM-LAB	0548455 F	4.00	4.00	
06	05	CHEM-LAB	0548519 F	5.00	5.00	
06	05	CHEM-LAB	0548660 F	12.50	12.50	
06	05	CHEM-LAB	0548663 F	12.50	12.50	
06	05	CHEM-LAB	0548213 F	5.75	5.75	
06	05	X-RAY	0524317 E	24.00	24.00	
06	05	X-RAY	0524401 E	28.00	28.00	
06	05	XRAY-PORTABLE-FILMS	0525082 E	8.00	8.00	
06	05	X-RAY	0525207 E	8.00	8.00	
06	05	ROOM BF		90.00	67.68	22.32
06	06	CHEM LAB	0548444 F	12.00	12.00	
06	06	CHEM-LAB	0548221 F	25.00CR	25.00CR	
06	06	B-M-R-LAB	0644006 F	5.00	5.00	
06	06	I V SOLUTION	14610 D	115.00	115.00	
06	06	MEDICATION	08754 D	23.10	23.10	
06	06	MEDICATION	08754 D	1.10	1.10	
06	06	MEDICATION	05650 D	39.95	39.95	
06	06	MEDICATION	20290 D	16.60	16.60	
06	06	MEDICATION	31040 D	3.50	3.50	
06	06	MEDICATION	15160 D	25.20	25.20	
06	06	MEDICATION	15160 D	3.60	3.60	
06	06	MEDICATION	15000 D	7.95	7.95	
06	06	MEDICATION	17625 D	102.00	102.00	
06	06	MEDICATION	13310 D	3.00	3.00	
06	06	SFT. LUMBAR PUNCTURE	0373674 G	.80	.80	

T 6 25M 1/65   PLEASE MAKE CHECKS PAYABLE TO THE MASSACHUSETTS GENERAL HOSPITAL   PAY LAST AMOUNT IN THIS COLUMN

✠

The single most important problem facing modern hospitals is cost. This cost can be analyzed in a variety of ways, most of them confusing and unhelpful. But the following points are clear:

First, the cost of hospitalization has skyrocketed. The average MGH patient today pays *per hour* what the average patient paid *per day* in 1925. Even as recently as 1940, a private patient could have his room for $10.25 per day; by 1964, it cost $50.10 per day; by 1969, $72.00–$110.00 per day. This staggering increase is continuing at the rate of 6 to 8 per cent per year. Each year for the past three, the MGH has had to raise its charges. Nor is the teaching hospital unique in its financial squeeze. All American hospitals are raising their charges at this same rate.

Second, hospitalization cost has increased much more rapidly than other goods and services in the economy. Medical care is the fastest-rising item in the consumer price index in recent years, and per-day hospital cost accounts for the largest proportion of this increase.*

Third, the individual contemplating hospitalization no longer worries much, in a direct way, about cost. Third-party payment has led to public apathy about hospital costs, and this is unwise—if for no other reason than the fact that most people have only one fourth to one third of their costs paid by insurance, a fact they discover late in the game.

Fourth, the often overlapping coverage of health in-

---

* Physicians' fees have also been rising faster than other items in the consumer price index. However, hospital costs have been nearly doubled in the past decade, while physicians' fees have increased 30 per cent.

surance permits some patients to make money from their hospitalization, while welfare reimbursements are always less than the true costs of care. In this situation, the hospital makes ends meet by overcharging private patients and their insurance companies to cover the welfare deficit—in the case of the MGH, roughly $10 a day overcharge.

Fifth, no single hospital stands alone in its financing problems, but rather is influenced by the activity or decline of other hospitals in the area. The decay of the Boston City Hospital, and its reduction in size to nearly half its earlier patient capacity, has created great pressure upon other Boston hospitals to take up the slack— by accepting precisely those patients on whom the hospital loses money, namely, patients covered by welfare. The decline of Boston's municipal, tax-supported hospital is similar to the decline of other such institutions in other American cities. In each case, the reasons behind the decline are political and financial, but the consequences are always the same—to pass on costs to insured patients, and make them augment insufficient tax funding for welfare. In the long run, of course, it all works out to the same thing: one can either pay the money in taxes or in higher health-insurance premiums. But in such a situation, it is probably more efficient to choose one or the other—and the trend unmistakably is toward universal health insurance in this country. Dr. John Knowles notes that many Americans are required by law to arrange insurance for their cars; why should they not also be required to arrange health insurance for themselves?

Sixth, lest private health insurance seem a financial panacea, one should note that private companies are often irrational in their payment procedures. For example, for many years one could not collect for certain treatments—such as the setting of fractures—unless one were admitted to the hospital, at least overnight. Thus a person who might easily receive therapy in the EW and be sent home had to be admitted in order to receive insurance coverage. This unnecessary admission raised the total cost of health care, and ultimately such increases are passed on to the consumer in the form of higher premiums. Some of these odd payment procedures have been changed, but not all.

Seventh, the American medical system in its full spectrum—from the private specialist's office to the municipal hospital wards—has never been able to structure the kind of competitive situation that encourages and rewards economies. Nor has American medicine tried. The American physician has been grossly irresponsible in nearly all matters relating to the cost of medical care. One can trace this irresponsibility quite directly to the American Medical Association.

For the past forty years, the American Medical Association has worked to the detriment of the patient in nearly every way imaginable; it is a pecularity of this organization that it has worked to the detriment of physicians, as well. Dr. James Howard Means has said: "Its ideology is very like that of the big labor unions . . . it has now set up a continuing political action committee quite like those of the fighting labor unions. Every attempt that has been made by liberally minded groups to improve medical care and make it more accessible . . . the AMA has attacked with ever increasing truculence. . . . They forget perhaps that medicine is for the people, not for the doctors. They need some enlightenment on this point."

The truculence of the AMA has been expensive. In terms of the modern-day cost of medical care, we may cite the following points. Beginning in 1930, it opposed voluntary health insurance, such as Blue Cross. In 1932, it opposed prepaid group-practice clinics. In 1933, it began a successful campaign to block the construction of new medical schools and limit enrollment in those already in existence. We now have a shortage of doctors. More recently, the AMA spent millions—probably no one knows exactly how many millions—to fight Medicare, a program that resulted in health benefits to 10 per cent of the population and vastly increased income to physicians. (Indeed, a good gauge of the AMA's shortsightedness can be gained by imagining the outcry from private doctors should anyone now try to repeal Medicare.) Further, the AMA has failed to take any strong stand on prescription pharmaceutical prices in this country, which nearly every objective observer regards as grossly inflated. And more insidiously, the AMA has permitted what may politely be called blind spots in

64

health care. The *Journal of the American Medical Association* refused to print a government study of combination-antibiotic drugs which concluded that many of these expensive medications are either worthless or dangerous; the AMA has still failed to condemn cigarette smoking despite overwhelming evidence that this habit, though profitable to certain industrial groups, is directly responsible for much disease, suffering, and medical expense in this country.

One can only conclude that the American Medical Association has not considered the interests of patients for forty years, or perhaps longer. On the basis of its record, it is opposed to both better and cheaper medical care. Its only commitment is to the doctor's bank account—and even then, it makes astonishing errors in judgment.

In 1967, in his inaugural address, Milford O. Rouse, the incoming president of the AMA, deplored the growing sentiment in this country that medical care was a right, not a privilege. His opinion was not well received by an angry public, and later presidents have been more circumspect in voicing their views. Nonetheless, it is customary for AMA presidents to travel about, speaking to groups of doctors, applauding what they call "the phenomenal growth of the health industry."

That growth cannot be questioned. Personal consumption expenditures for medical care rose from $7.5 billion in 1948 to over $27 billion in 1965, and more than $50 billion in 1968. By 1975, it is expected to reach

$100 billion or more. This is the sort of news to make a Wall Street broker squeal with delight. But medicine is a service, not an industry, and one really ought to look at it differently.

In fact, the United States spends more of its gross national product (6.2 per cent) on medical care than any other country in the world; it spends a larger absolute sum than any other country in the world. Yet by most objective standards of health—infant mortality, life expectancy, and so on—it is far from the leader.

Other countries are doing better, and most of them have some form of socialized medicine. The United States is extraordinarily backward in this respect. However, many clear-headed American observers have looked at European socialized systems and have come away shaking their heads; and there is a widespread doubt whether any European system can be adapted to this country. Very likely, America will have to work out its own system. The combination of group insurance with a group-practice system (essentially the system at Kaiser and others) seems a feasible, economical, and practical method, acceptable both to doctors and patients.

Without question, the notion of the doctor as a legitimate fee-for-service entrepreneur, making his fortune from the misfortunes of his patients, is old fashioned, distasteful, and doomed. It is only a question of time.

✠

Ultimately, however, it is not useful to lay blame, whether on physicians, health-insurance administrators, politicians, or an apathetic public. For they all seem to share a common blindness—a total failure to understand why hospital costs are rising. In 1967, the average cost of a hospital room in America increased 15 per cent. What is happening?

The per-day room charge is the largest single item in the hospital bill. There are many ways to break down this charge—as many ways as there are accountants—but the clearest is the following.

In 1969, the cost of a semi-private room at the MGH was $70.00. Breaking this down, we find:

PER-DAY ROOM CHARGE: $70.00

Utilities, housekeeping, maintenance, plus business offices ("hotel expense")	$ 6.96
Food and special diets	5.82
Nursing	18.42
Labs, records, house staff, X rays, and pharmacy	28.80
Overcharge (to cover welfare debts)	10.00
Total	$70.00

Now this breakdown contradicts one of the oldest complaints about hospitals, as quoted in a national magazine: "My work puts me in contact with hotels and hotel management and I *know* that a good hotel can give you a beautiful room for $30.00 a day, with three meals, and make a profit and pay taxes. And yet any hospital, which doesn't pay *any* taxes, operates in the red for $65.00 a day. I say it must be poor administration."

If the analogy were true, the conclusion would be correct. But the hospital is not a hotel—and in any case, its "hotel" costs are quite reasonable at $6.96 a day; this is approximately half the cost of a decent motel room in Boston. The charge of $5.82 for food, or approximately $1.95 a meal, is equally reasonable, especially when one considers that as a restaurant the hospital must provide an extraordinary range of services, including some eighty special diets.

The *true* hospital costs—the expenses incurred in a hospital but not in a hotel—are, on the other hand, very high. They account for 82 per cent of the total per-day room charge. And the question, really, is whether these charges are reducible. No sensible businessman would bother to try to get his hotel and food costs below thirteen dollars a day; if there is to be a decrease in costs, it must come from the non-hotel charges.

These in turn largely reflect the increased technological capacity of the hospital. Mr. O'Connor's example is a case in point: most of the tests performed on him were not available in 1925, when he could have had his room for one twenty-fifth of what it cost him today. The maintenance of this new technological capability costs money—and to a large extent, in medicine as in educa-

68

tion, law enforcement, sanitation, and a variety of other services, you get what you pay for. If you are going to enter a high-quality acute-care facility that has six employees (most of them non-physicians) for every patient, and if you are going to pay these employees a decent wage, then your care will be expensive.* If you are going to purchase technological hardware, maintain it, and keep it up to date, this costs money. If you are going to keep the hospital in continuous operation twenty-four hours a day, three hundred sixty-five days a year, this costs money.

All this becomes clear in the instance of a simple procedure such as a chest X ray. A private radiologist in his office will perform this for you at one half or one third of what the hospital charges. His charge largely reflects the fact that his unit can operate on an eight-hour day and a forty-hour week; other costs, such as equipment and supplies, are the same. In medicine today—as in every other industry—people are more expensive than anything else. Sixty-three per cent of the hospital budget now goes to the salaries and benefits of employees. And much of the rise in hospital costs is directly attributable to the demand of these employees that they not be personally forced to subsidize the health business by accepting wages incommensurate with similar jobs in

---

* All this is sometimes easier to see if it is taken out of the hospital setting. If a man had to hire six secretaries for an eight-hour day, at $2.50 an hour, it would cost him $120.00 a day. If a man had to hire two gardeners at $4.00 an hour, for a single eight-hour day, it would still cost him $64.00 a day.

other industries. Their demands are justified; most employees are still underpaid. Their salaries will increase in the future.

✠

One cannot, however, fairly claim that hospitals are superbly efficient. Especially in a teaching hospital, attention to cost in the medical, non-hotel sector is less central than one would like it to be. One can argue about whether too many tests are ordered, and the argument can continue endlessly. But certainly, when physicians who order these tests don't know what patients are charged for them, eyebrows must go up. In general, doctors tend to operate on a "spare no expense" philosophy which will, eventually, need to be tempered.

But, more fundamentally, the present cost structure of the hospital seems to lead to a rather old-fashioned conclusion: no one should go there unless he absolutely has to.

If a diagnostic procedure can be done on an ambulatory, out-patient basis, it should be; if a series of tests and X rays can be done outside the hospital, they should be. No one should be admitted unless his care absolutely depends upon being inside the hospital; no one should be admitted unless he requires the hour-to-hour facilities of the house staff, the nursing staff, and the laboratories.

For decades, admission to the hospital was necessary

because there was no other facility available. For a large segment of the population, care was either given in the hospital, or not at all; and the hospital's clinic system was a poor compromise, with hordes of patients being brought in to wait hours—sometimes literally days—to have relatively brief tests performed.

There is hope that the satellite clinics will help solve the problem; one study of a satellite clinic in Boston reported that there were fewer hospital admissions as a result of the clinic's work.

In any case, alternative facilities must be found, because it is unlikely that hospital costs will ever go down. The best anyone can hope to do in the foreseeable future is stabilize them somewhere in the neighborhood of $100.00 a day. This makes the hospital an expensive place—but it has its uses, and indeed will be an economically tolerable place, if it is used appropriately.

PETER LUCHESI

At 3:15 p.m., the emergency ward was notified that a patient was being transferred in from an outlying hospital: a young man with a nearly severed arm resulting from an industrial accident.

He arrived an hour later and was seen first by Dr. Hopkins, the triage officer, who ordered him sent to OR 1. The surgical residents, Drs. Eugene Appel and Terry Mixter, were called to examine the new patient.

He was twenty-two years old, of medium height and muscular build, looked quite pale, and was speaking weakly. His left hand was bandaged and splinted. An intravenous line had been inserted in his right arm, but it had infiltrated. There was also a bandage over his chin.

75

The bandages were removed and a new intravenous line started. He had a moderately deep two-inch laceration in his chin; the medical student, Sue Rosenthal, was called to suture it. Meanwhile, Appel and Mixter turned their attention to the injured arm.

Three inches above the left wrist the forearm had been mashed. Bones stuck out at all angles; reddish areas of muscle with silver fascial coats were exposed in many places. The entire arm above the injury was badly swollen, but the hand was still normal size, although it looked shrunken and atrophic in comparison. The color of the hand was deep blue-gray.

Carefully, Appel picked up the hand, which flopped loosely at the wrist. He checked pulses and found none below the elbow. He touched the fingers of the hand with a pin and asked if Luchesi could feel it; results were confusing, but there appeared to be some loss of sensation. He asked if the patient could move any of his fingers; he could not.

Meanwhile the orthopedic resident, Dr. Robert Hussey, arrived and examined the hand. He concluded that both bones in the forearm, the radius and ulna, were broken, and suggested the hand be elevated; he proceeded to do this.

Outside the door to the room, one of the admitting men stopped Appel. "Are you going to take it, or try to keep it?"

"Hell, we're going to keep it," Appel said. "That's a good hand."

The patient was started on two grams of cephalothin antibiotic intravenously, and was given more tetanus toxoid. He had received pain medication at the other hospital, and so far had not requested more.

As a workmen's compensation case, the operation would be done by private surgeons: Dr. Hugh Chandler for orthopedics, Dr. Ashby Moncure for general surgery. At 5:15, Moncure arrived and looked at the hand, satisfied himself that it was indeed viable, and put the patient on call for the operating room. He also called Chandler and summarized the case: "It's a circumferential crush injury to the left hand with compound fracture of both radius and ulna. Innervation and arterial supply look pretty good."

Meantime, the portable X-ray machine was brought in to take a chest film, and two views of the injured hand. The medical student finished suturing the chin laceration. Moncure came back to check that a sample had been sent to the blood bank. He then went off to try to hasten scheduling for the operating room.

At 5:30, the patient complained for the first time of pain in his hand. The surgeons were debating what pain medication to give him when a nurse came in to say the patient was on call to the OR and would get pre-operative medication. He received atropine, Nembutal, and demerol, which settled the question of pain medication.

Dr. Hussey, looking at the now-elevated hand, concluded that it appeared a little better; the color had improved. He wrapped the injured area in soft gauze, and went off to the X-ray unit to examine the films. He went directly to the residents' reading room, a cubicle with lighted, frosted glass walls for examining X rays. The resident was busy reading other films; Hussey went back into the developing room, past signs which forbade him to do so, to get Luchesi's films. A female technician scolded him; he said he was in a hurry.

He gave the films to the radiologic resident, who put them up and dictated: "Unit number zero zero six, AP and lateral of the left forearm. There is a transverse fracture of the radius in the distal third, as well as the ulna, period. Numerous fragments of bone are scattered around the fracture site, period. Considerable soft tissue swelling . . ." Here he stopped, realizing Hussey was impatient. "Chest film normal," he dictated, and gave them all to Hussey, who returned to the patient and supervised his transport to the operating rooms on the third floor.

It was now six o'clock. The operation was scheduled for 6:15, at which time on the OR blackboard was written:

RM 7   PVT. SERVICE   SEVERED ARM   MONCURE/CHANDLER

In the operating room, Dr. Brian Dalton, the first of three anesthetists who would work during the six-hour procedure, was administering an axillary block, injecting lidocaine (a novocaine-like drug) deep into the armpit, to dull, during the preparation, sensation in the nerves that ran out to the hand. While this was being done, Moncure discussed the operation: "What we're going to do here is stabilize his bones, and then deal with soft tissues as need be. I think we'll find a lot of crush damage to muscle bellies, particularly flexors, but intact vessels and nerves." He observed that while clinically there was questionable nerve damage, a crush injury could produce this without any actual cutting of nerve fibers; under such circumstances the damage was probably fully reversible.

At 6:10, while the axillary block was being administered, Hugh Chandler, the orthopedic surgeon, arrived and looked at the X rays. He said that he would stabilize one bone, the radius, and worry about the other, the ulna, later. Moncure was outside the OR, scrubbing according to the MGH version of the ritual: three minutes of washing to the elbow with a hard bristle brush, using orange sticks to clean under the nails, followed by a dunking to the elbows in an alcohol-germicidal solution. When he finished his scrub he came in, put on a pair of sterile rubber gloves, and began to wash the arm with a safety soap and alcohol. The nerve block was beginning to take effect, and it was possible to move the arm less gently without hurting the patient.

The patient was still awake, but dazed. He stared at his arm curiously, as if it did not belong to him. Moncure asked him how it had happened. Peter Luchesi explained that he had been working in a private shipyard and a boom had fallen on him. It weighed seven hundred pounds and it had struck his shoulder glancingly, knocking him overboard. But as he fell, the boom had somehow landed on his hand, leaving him dangling over the side, with his hand pinned down. This was just after lunch. The other workmen were not on the boat, so Luchesi had managed to get back up on the deck alone, and attempted to lift the boom. He could not do it without help. Fifteen minutes passed before the others arrived and were able to lift the boom.

He delivered the entire story in a monotone, while he stared at his hand. Moncure asked him how it felt now, and he said it was beginning to hurt again. As the surgeons began to drape the injured arm with sterile cloths, which entailed considerable manipulation of the hand, he complained more. The axillary block was not working well. With all preparation made, now was the time to produce general anesthesia.

Dalton, the anesthetist, leaned over Luchesi and said: "I'm going to put this mask over your face. You'll breathe only oxygen. Then I'll give you an injection that will make you fall asleep. Don't worry about a thing, just breathe and relax."

Luchesi nodded. The mask was put over his face and he breathed, staring up at Dalton, who proceeded to inject pentathol intravenously. Luchesi blinked once and closed his eyes. He was sleeping soundly, but would continue to do so for only a few minutes. Then he would wake up, unless more pentothal, or a different anesthetic, was administered.

Luchesi was fed pure oxygen for several moments, to be sure he was fully oxygenated. Then Dalton injected succinylcholine, a substance that paralyzes the entire body—including respiratory muscles—briefly. He removed the mask, opened the mouth, squirted a jet of cocaine down the throat to anesthetize the windpipe and prevent reflex coughing, and slipped a tube down the mouth into the windpipe. This provided a direct channel from the mouth into the windpipe and lungs, and prevented a major cause of death from anesthesia, namely, vomiting up of food from the stomach and blockage of the windpipe with this material.

The entire process of intubation took only a few seconds. Once intubated, Luchesi was fed oxygen and nitrous oxide, a mild anesthetic. Alone, nitrous oxide would not provide sufficiently deep anesthesia to permit surgery, but the axillary block was also helping. When it wore off, halothane, a more potent gas, would be added.

The operation began shortly before seven. There were seven people in the operating room at that time. Five were scrubbed: Moncure and Chandler, sitting on one side of the outstretched hand; Dr. Charles Brennan, an orthopedic resident, and Steven Kroll, a medical student, on the other side; and the scrub nurse, standing with two trays of instruments at her fingertips. Also in the room but not scrubbed were the anesthetist and the circulating nurse.

Around the hand, it was tight quarters. The scrub

nurse first pinned sterile towels across the backs of Moncure and Chandler; this was because the uppermost portions of their backs, where the sterile gowns were tied, were unsterile, and she did not want to touch them by accident.

In general, the operating room is divided conceptually into "clean" and "dirty" areas. The operative field, meaning the exposed area of skin which has been shaved, scrubbed—and generally covered with plastic—is clean. The rest of the patient, covered with sterile drapes, is dirty. The fronts of the surgeons are clean; their backs are dirty. Anything above the level of the table is clean; anything below is dirty, and surgeons never let their hands fall to their sides. Hands, scrubbed and rubber-covered, are clean; faces, capped and masked, are dirty, and it is poor form to get one's face too close to the operative field or to touch one's mask with one's gloved hand.

The first incision was made over the underside of the wrist, just back from the thumb. The object was to find and locate the radial artery in that area. Moncure and Chandler discussed their procedure as they went, and agreed to find and evaluate the principal structures first: the radial and ulnar arteries, which run toward thumb and little finger respectively; the radial and ulnar nerves, which run with the arteries; and the median nerve, which enters the hand at mid-wrist.

As they began work, they found that the crush injury, with its hemorrhage and swelling of tissues, made identification of structures difficult. Five minutes into the operation, the radial artery was accidentally nicked. A fine, thin stream of blood spurted up in a foot-long arc. This was quickly clamped, and Moncure sewed it up with a small needle, perhaps no larger than twice the size of a typewriter parenthesis mark, and the operation proceeded. Moncure isolated the radial artery for a distance of several inches through the wrist. Everyone commented on the fact that pulsations through the artery were not as strong as they would like. The artery was flushed with heparin to prevent clotting further along its course in the hand.

At 7:20, Dr. Leslie Ottinger, another surgeon, entered the operating room. He had been working next door in OR 8 for six hours, repairing a crush injury to a man's thigh. Moncure, without looking up, said to Ottinger: "Were your vessels intact?"

"No," Ottinger said. "The femoral artery and vein were completely crushed. They were separated by three centimeters."

"How's he doing now?"

"Fine," Ottinger said, "if he stays open." He watched the dissection of the hand for some moments. "You find the radial artery yet?"

"We nicked it," Moncure said.

"Well, that's a good way to find it," Ottinger said, and left.

As the operation progressed, Moncure noted that the surgical field was more bloody. He felt the radial artery

83

and concluded that it was pulsating more fully now.

By eight o'clock, the contrast between the area of surgical dissection and the area of crush injury was clear. One was clean and smooth, nicely exposed, bleeding very little; the other was mashed and oozing blood. Moncure, still working, glanced up at the clock and said: "Ottinger and I had a squash game for eight o'clock. We both ended up here. That'll teach us."

The operation itself proceeded slowly, impeded by the difficulty of identifying structures within the injured area. When damaged, a tendon, vein, and nerve can all look remarkably alike, but identification must be made with certainty. Nearly any vein in the body can be cut without consequence; to cut a tendon is an irritation, but not irreparable; to cut an important nerve is a disaster of major proportions.

Eventually all the structures were identified. All were found to be intact except for the ulnar artery, which was completely torn. The muscular coat of the artery was in spasm, pinching it off; the ends were clipped for the time being, and Chandler took over to begin work on the bones.

His first decision was to shorten the left arm by half an inch. This was necessary because there was a fragment missing from the ulna, and both radius and ulna had to be the same length. Also, shortening would make repair of tendons easier. He pointed out that this shortening would not be noticeable to the patient or anybody looking at him.

84

He began by filing the ends of the radius smooth and then joining them together with a vitalium plate, made of an alloy of cobalt, chromium, and molybdenum. It is electrically neutral and well tolerated by bone and the tissues around it. Screwing the plate onto the bone was difficult; it was not completed until 10:30.

Meanwhile, the anesthetist had been making some changes. "The axillary block has worn off by now," he said. "So we're supplementing the nitrous oxide with halothane in low concentrations. If he needs more for pain, we'll raise the halothane." He indicated that he could judge the need for anesthetic by watching the patient who, while not waking up, would become restless and would breathe irregularly if he was "too light."

"The idea," he said, "is to give the minimal anesthetic necessary to do the job, and to give it in such a way that the patient wakes up as soon as possible after the operation."

After Chandler repaired the radius, Moncure resumed vascular and soft-tissue reconstruction. He first reexamined the radial artery and decided it was not flowing as well as it should, as judged by squeezing the artery wall and feeling the pulsations. To make certain it was clear, he called for a small Fogarty catheter. This is a small, flexible tube with an inflatable rubber bulb at one tip. From the opposite end, water can be injected into the tube, and the bulb will expand. Thus the catheter can be inserted down an artery, and the bulb inflated within the artery. It can then be drawn back while in-

flated, and in doing so, it will clean out the inner wall of
the artery, removing clots and other obstructions.

The Fogarty catheter is a relatively new device, named
for its inventor, a surgeon at Stanford Medical Center.
The discussion that ensued is typical of medicine in the
modern day. So many developments and products are
becoming available that it is difficult for anyone to keep
track.

Moncure: "Get me the smallest Fogarty you have."

The circulating nurse came back with one. "This is a
number four."

Moncure: "Let's have a look at it." He removed it
from its plastic container; it looked too large. "Are you
sure you haven't got something smaller?"

Scrub nurse to circulating nurse: "I know we have a
six, at least."

"But a six is larger than a four," the circulating nurse
said. She said it hesitantly, since numbers to designate
sizes do not always run the same way. For instance,
urinary catheters and nasogastric tubes run in proportion to size—a number fourteen is larger than a number
twelve. But needles and sutures run in the opposite
direction: an eighteen is much larger than a twenty-
one needle.

"Well, see if there's something smaller."

It turned out there wasn't. Moncure meantime had
made a small cut in the artery wall, and had found he
could slip in the number four Fogarty without difficulty.
He inflated the bulb, drew back, and found that the

subsequent pulse was much improved. He sewed the cut shut, and felt the pulse. "Bounding now," he said.

He directed his attention to the ulnar artery, which had been completely severed by the injury. The ulnar was smaller than the radial artery; it was about the size of a pencil lead. As Moncure began to sew the ends together with fine sutures, he said, "Microsurgery. Watchmaking." It was now 11:30. He sewed it quite quickly, and the remainder of the operation, which dealt with larger structures, went rapidly. The tendons that had been torn were resewn. A heavy pin was run down the hollow interior of the ulna. By 12:30, the surgeons began to close.

It had been known from the outset that the wound area could not be completely closed. The tissues were damaged and swollen; to pull the skin tight across it would compress the arteries and cut off circulation to the hand, negating all the efforts of surgery. The incision was therefore only partially closed, with an area of the inner wrist left open. This area was expected to close by itself, to a degree, and to scar over for the remainder; after four or five days, they would re-evaluate the area to consider skin grafting. The surgeons' major concern was infection. It was decided to continue the patient on cephalothin.

The operation was finished at one in the morning. The patient awoke in the operating room and was taken to the recovery room. For the first twenty-four hours, he was kept heavily sedated, but by the third day his pain was considerably less. Two weeks later he was discharged from the hospital. Two months later, on an office visit, Moncure found that the patient had essentially full function and sensation in the nearly severed hand.

✠

The growth of modern surgery within the hospital is chiefly attributable to three factors. The first is the discovery of anesthesia. The second is the introduction of aseptic techniques. And the third, much more recent, is the improved medical understanding of the patient, with attendant improvements in pre-operative and, especially, post-operative care.

Consider anesthesia first. One hundred and three years before Peter Luchesi's hand was sewn back on, John C. Warren wrote: "Surgery has ceased to be the spectacular occupation it once was." It is impossible to miss the regret in his words, but he did not mean it regretfully, for he was talking about the difference anesthesia had made to surgery.

It is hard to imagine now how ghastly, horrible, and hasty surgery was before anesthesia. In Warren's own recollection:

In the case of amputation, it was the custom to bring the patient into the operating room and place him upon the table. [The surgeon] would stand with his hands behind his back and would say to the patient, "Will you have your leg off, or

88

will you not have it off?" If the patient lost courage and said "No," he was at once carried back to his bed in the ward. If, however, he said "Yes," he was immediately taken firmly in hand by a number of strong assistants and the operation went on regardless of whatever he might say thereafter.

Relief from pain was not the only benefit of anesthesia. Equally important was muscular relaxation, which prior to ether was produced as follows: "In the case of a dislocated hip, where it was necessary to effect complete muscular relaxation, an enema of tobacco was freely administered, and while the victim was reduced to the last stages of collapse from nicotine poisoning the dislocated femur was forced back into its place."

One might expect this deplorable state of affairs would lead surgeons to search for ways to kill pain and to be constantly alert for new drugs that might accomplish the job. But in fact this did not happen: pain-killing drugs were known for forty years before they were applied to surgery. If, as Poincaré says, discovery favors the prepared mind, doctors must be counted strangely unprepared. Briefly, the story is this:

Nitrous oxide was isolated by the English chemist Joseph Priestley in 1772. Around 1800, another Englishman, Humphrey Davy, experimented with the gas, noted its exhilarating and pain-killing properties and suggested it might be used in surgery. The suggestion was ignored. Instead, "laughing gas" became a popular form of amusement on both sides of the Atlantic. In 1818, ether was found to have the same effect as nitrous oxide. Soon thereafter, "ether frolics" came into vogue, especially among medical students and house officers—indeed, a whole generation of young doctors toyed with immortality, but missed the point. The observation was repeatedly made that one could bruise himself while under ether and have no recollection of the cause later, but no one connected the phenomenon to surgical applications. The blindness of these young men is sobering. (It also makes one think more highly of Alexander Fleming, whose culture dishes, contaminated with mold, might have been thrown out. One wonders how many hundreds of researchers before him had seen penicillin-producing molds, and had attached no significance to them.)

To make matters worse, when ether was finally used successfully in surgery by two men in 1842—Crawford W. Long in Georgia and Elijah Pope in New York— neither publicized his work widely, and their work had no impact on future events.

In 1844, Horace Wells, a Hartford dentist, painlessly extracted a tooth with nitrous oxide. He immediately communicated this news to a former dentist, then a Harvard medical student, William T. G. Morton. Morton in turn obtained permission for Wells to come to Boston and demonstrate anesthesia before the class of Dr. John C. Warren at the MGH. Wells did this soon after, but apparently did not obtain sufficiently deep anesthesia with nitrous oxide (which is, in any case, not a powerful anesthetic). At the crucial moment, the patient screamed; the students hissed; Wells slunk off in disgrace.

The idea of painless operation was abandoned as hopeless fantasy by all except Morton, who later met a chemist named Charles T. Jackson. Jackson suggested the use of ether instead of nitrous oxide; Morton found that it worked and himself approached Warren for a chance to demonstrate the method publicly. It is to Warren's credit that, despite a resounding failure only a short time before, he agreed to a second trial under his auspices. This occurred on October 16, 1846, in the hospital amphitheater under the Bulfinch Dome.

It must have been a strange scene. Morton arrived late, permitting some jokes about a last minute failure of nerve. The patient, a man with a tumor under the jaw, sat in a straight-back chair, facing Warren and the assembled students, all wearing frock coats. Also in the room were articles then considered fit decoration for an operating theater: a skeleton, a large marble statue of Apollo, and a mummy from Thebes. A photographer was also present, but according to a newspaper account, "the sight of blood so unnerved him that he was obliged to retire."

Apparently the photographer was the only person to experience pain that day, for the patient underwent deep anesthesia, made no sound during surgery, and when he awoke, reported that he had felt nothing. Dr. Warren, then sixty-eight years old, turned with tears in his eyes to the audience and said, "Gentlemen, this is no humbug."*

News of the operation spread with extraordinary rapidity. The first English ether operation was done some ten weeks later; it was performed by the noted surgeon Robert Liston, who first announced skeptically, "We are going to try a Yankee dodge to make men insensible." Although the anesthetic worked, Liston operated with his customary speed, single-handedly amputating the leg at the thigh in exactly twenty-eight seconds.

✠

The first important effect of anesthesia was to increase the number of operations performed. The second was to lengthen the time of operation: the split-second showmanship of Liston and many others became obsolete

* Morton, who anesthetized Warren's patient, attempted to exploit his discovery for financial gain. He labeled the ether "letheon" and tried to disguise its characteristic smell with various aromatic oils, hoping no one would discover it was only ether. The ploy failed and even the name was dropped when Oliver Wendell Holmes suggested that "anesthetic" would be a better word.

Undaunted, Morton then petitioned Congress for an award for his discovery. The sum of one hundred thousand dollars was suggested, but he never received it; almost immediately a Southern senator put forward a claim in the name of Crawford Long, and Charles Jackson, the Boston chemist, entered one of his own. Debate raged until the outbreak of the Civil War turned the attention of Congress to other matters.

The aftermath of all this is depressing. Horace Wells, the Hartford dentist, went insane, was jailed for throwing acid at two girls, and committed suicide while in prison. Charles Jackson also went insane and died in an asylum. William Morton died a forgotten pauper on a park bench at the age of forty-nine.

overnight, and new standards of meticulous skill sprang up.

But problems were far from ended. Difficulty with infection remained for many years afterward, until Joseph Lister in Scotland formulated his antiseptic methods.

Within the hospital, cross-infection was common-place for all patients. But surgical patients, in the absence of sterile operating techniques, were particularly prone to infection, and one effect of increasing the duration of operations was to increase the opportunity for bacterial contamination of the wound. Thus, in the decades after the introduction of anesthesia, the chief cause of surgical mortality was infection.*

There was confusion about infection caused by cross-contamination, from wound infection, and from decomposition of dead tissue within the wound. In the absence of clear understanding, hospital infections—termed "hospitalism"—were generally attributed to gen-

---

* The great majority of surgical incisions became infected afterward and surgeons spoke favorably of "laudable pus" in the wound. But as Edward D. Churchill has said, "To intimate that surgeons before Lister expected all wounds to suppurate and pour forth 'laudable pus' is to underestimate the intelligence of generations of shrewd observers over the course of centuries. . . . Hippocrates taught that dead flesh in a wound must turn to pus, but Theodoric as well as Mondeville [two medieval surgeons] expected *incised* wounds, in which dead tissue is customarily minimal, to heal without suppuration as a matter of course. In Lister's own century, at the Battle of Waterloo, it was generally agreed among English surgeons that if the edges of clean-cut saber wounds were drawn together by adhesive straps, healing would be accomplished without suppuration. Listerism could not, nor did it pretend to, eliminate suppuration arising in contaminated dead tissue. . . . The principle of excision of dead tissue (debridement) as the initial step in wound management finally emerged in the 1914–1918 war."

eral environmental causes. The location of the hospital was deemed crucial.

The Massachusetts General was built on reclaimed land. It was noted that during the summer "the neighborhood was rendered offensive and unwholesome by emanations from the flats and newly made land." In 1875, the Board of Consultation recommended to hospital trustees that "no more buildings should be erected upon the land adjacent to the present wards because of improper (land) filling. . . . At some future time, it will be for the best interest of the hospital if the buildings should be given up and a new site selected, one more fitted to the purposes of a hospital than the present one is now or ever can be."

The date of this comment, 1875, is significant, for Listerian antisepsis had been introduced six years before to the MGH by staff members who had visited the Scottish innovator's hospital in Edinburgh. Antisepsis was not widely accepted in this country, however, for nearly thirty years afterward. Instead, environmental arguments continued—despite the fact that Lister had halved infection rates in a hospital that was built on the site of a makeshift cemetery in which thousands of cholera victims had been shallowly buried only a decade previously.

It took less than three months for anesthesia to gain wide acceptance in medicine. It took more than thirty years for antisepsis to be accepted. Why? Both discoveries addressed themselves to equally important prob-

lems—if anything, infection was an even greater problem than pain. And both techniques, though primitive,
certainly worked. What accounts for the difference in
speed of acceptance?

Scientific understanding is not part of it. At the time
the two innovations were proposed, neither could be explained. And though we now understand antisepsis,
we still cannot explain why anesthetic gases kill pain.

Nor is diffusion of information a problem. News of
antisepsis spread as quickly as news of anesthesia. Lister's techniques were widely and hotly debated in every
Western country.

Rather, the answer seems to lie with medicine's capacity to deal with individuals versus groups. Anesthesia
was dramatic, it produced a positive effect, and it could
be seen working in the individual. On the other hand,
antisepsis was passive, not dramatic, and negative in
the sense that it tried to *prevent* an effect, not produce
one. It was common in the early days of antisepsis for
a skeptical surgeon to half-heartedly try the lengthy, ex-
asperating techniques on one or two patients, find that
the patients still became infected, and generalize from
this experience to conclude the system was worthless.
Nor can one really hold this against them, for a modern
understanding of individual and group effects—the notion, for example, of a "controlled clinical trial" in all
its statistical ramifications—is very recent indeed.

Nonetheless, antisepsis eventually became accepted
in principle and thereafter followed a string of con-

tributions to sterile operative technique. William S. Halsted, the Johns Hopkins surgeon, is credited with introducing rubber gloves for surgery in 1898. Special gowns to replace street clothes came at the turn of the century. Masks were not common until the late 1920's.

Ultimately, antibiotics provided the final powerful tool. Thus, in the space of a century, surgical mortality, which was generally 80 per cent at the time of the Civil War, was cut to 45 per cent by Listerian methods, and slowly cut even further in ensuing years, until it is now about 3 per cent in most hospitals.

Ways to reduce the percentage to zero are being explored. In recent years, the evolved ritual of timed scrubs, sterile gowns, rubber gloves, and masks has been criticized. Various studies have indicated that scrubbing does not clean the skin, but just loosens the bacteria on the hands, making them more mobile; that one quarter of all gloves have holes in them; that modern gowns are permeable to bacteria, especially if they become wet (as they often do in the course of operation); that doorways sealing off operating rooms do not prevent spread of bacteria but serve as collecting places for them. Such studies are too conflicting at present to see a clear trend, but it is likely that the ritual will be strongly modified in coming years.

Surgeons themselves tend to be almost complacent about the studies, largely because post-operative infection is no longer a major problem. In fact, the most common early, immediate, direct cause of death from surgery is not the operation but the anesthesia.

One wonders why this was not always so, especially in view of early methods for administering ether, by use of a cone-shaped sponge. J. C. Warren recalls that during the Civil War period:

These men, many of whom had become inured both to fighting and to a free use of alcohol, were not favorable subjects for the administration of ether, and I have still a vivid recollection of my efforts as a student and as house pupil at the hospital [1865–6] to etherize these patients. "Going under ether" in those days was no trifling ordeal and often was suggestive of the scrimmage of a football team rather than the quiet decorum which should surround the operating table. No preliminary treatment was thought necessary, except possibly to avoid the use of food for a certain time previous to the administration. Patients came practically as they were to the operating table and had to take their chances. They were usually etherized at the top of the staircase on a little chair outside the operating theater, as there was no room existing for this purpose at the time. In the struggle which ensued, I can recall often being forced against the bannisters with nothing but a thin rail to protect me from a fall down three flights. But however powerful the patient might be, the man behind the sponge came out victorious and the panting subject was carried triumphantly into the operating room by the house pupil and attendant.

Although the method of induction was primitive, it was not very dangerous. Profound anesthesia was difficult to accomplish and serious complications, Warren says, "were not commonly encountered."

Thus in a sense surgery has come a full circle, from the time when anesthesia opened new horizons to the time when anesthesia provides a serious hazard to operation. It is the kind of ironic twist that one frequently encounters in medical history.

A classic example of the full circle is the story of appendicitis. This is a very old disease—Egyptian mummies have been found who died of it—but it was never accurately described until 1886.

During most of the nineteenth century, surgeons were well aware of diseases which produced pain and pus in the right lower quadrant of the abdomen. Some attempts were even made to operate for the condition, by draining the abscess. But results were not encouraging and in 1874 the English surgeon Sir John Erickson said that the abdomen was "forever shut from the intrusion of the wise and humane surgeon." Note that pain was not a consideration here—surgical anesthesia was nearly thirty years old. Rather it was the fact that pus collections in the abdomen were not understood and did not appear to be helped by surgical intervention.

Twelve years later, an MGH pathologist named Reginald H. Fitz, who had traveled in Europe and studied under the great German pathologist Rudolf Virchow, published the results of an intensive study of 466 cases of "typhlitis" and "perityphlitic abscess," as the disease processes were then rather vaguely called. Fitz concluded

98

that what the surgeon found at operation—a large area of inflamed bowel and widespread pus in the abdominal cavity—had resulted from an initial, small infection in the appendix. By describing "appendicitis," he created, in effect, a new disease.

The new disease was not readily accepted by the medical profession. Nor was Fitz's assertion that proper treatment required operation *before* rupture, instead of afterward. Today the idea of "operative intervention" is commonplace, but in Fitz's day surgery was generally the last resort, not the first.

Even after his clinical description of appendicitis was accepted, the surgical treatment remained a matter of dispute. In many hospitals, appendectomy was considered a bizarre procedure of questionable value. In 1897, when Harvey Cushing was a house officer at Johns Hopkins (after having interned at MGH and having seen several appendectomies performed), he diagnosed appendicitis in himself. He had great difficulty convincing his colleagues to operate; both Halsted and Osler advised against it. Finally, however, the surgeons gave in and agreed to do the procedure. Cushing did all the rest: he admitted himself to the hospital, performed the admission physical examination on himself, diagrammed the abdominal findings, wrote his own pre-operative and post-operative orders. It was said that he would have performed the operation himself as well, had he been able to devise a way to do so.

In the next few years, appendicitis became not only

an acceptable but a fashionable disease; in 1902, it was diagnosed in King Edward VII of England, who was operated on for the condition. This signaled the onset of a great vogue for diagnosis and surgical treatment of appendicitis.

As a reasonably safe, reasonably simple abdominal operation, it encouraged surgeons to be more daring in exploring this body cavity. Their encouragement was not without its drawbacks, however: surgeons were so enthusiastic that nearly every bellyache was likely to receive an operation, and there sprang up a vogue for removal of ovaries and tubes in women, along with the appendix. The end result of this was the institution of quality control checks on surgical procedures, through the "tissue committees" headed by pathologists.

Dr. Francis D. Moore has said: "[Fitz] was a student of pathology telling the surgeons to do more operations. . . . How ironical it was that within thirty years it was to be the pathologists who applied the brakes to a surgical profession that was running wild with the operation for appendicitis."

Remembering Mr. O'Connor's case, it may be well to go into some of the differences, and some misconceptions regarding the relationship of surgeons and internists. The two groups have never been too congenial. Traditionally, physicians have considered themselves more intellectual than surgeons. Descendants of Hippocrates, they look down upon surgeons as descendants of barbers. Surgeons, on the other hand, see themselves as action-oriented and regard internists as procrastinators, unwilling and unable to take action.

Temperamentally and philosophically, the two groups are at loggerheads. At mealtimes in the doctors' dining room, medical and surgical house officers can be heard berating each other about the care their respective patients have received. The surgeons say that an internist will sit hapless by the bedside and watch a patient die; the internists say that the surgeon will cut anything that moves. Most of this talk represents a time-honored outlet for black humor, but there is a long history of genuine conflict.

Dr. Paul S. Russell quotes the surgeon Sir Heneage Ogilvie in a most revealing passage:

A surgeon conducting a difficult case is like the skipper of an ocean-going yacht. He knows the port he must make but he cannot foresee the course of the journey. . . . The physician's task is more comparable to that of the golfer. . . . If he judges the direction and the wind right, estimates each lie correctly, finds the right club for each shot and uses it successfully, he will get an eagle or a birdie. If he makes a mistake he will make a poor score but he will get there in the end. The ground will not split beneath his feet, the game will not change suddenly from golf to bull-fighting.

That was written in 1948. Six hundred years earlier, the French surgeon Henri de Mondeville set down his reasons for considering surgery superior to medicine:

Surgery is undoubtedly superior to medicine for the following reasons: 1. Surgery cures more complicated maladies, toward which medicine is helpless. 2. Surgery cures diseases that cannot be cured by any other means, not by themselves, not by nature, nor by medicine. Medicine indeed never cures a disease so evidently that one could say that the cure is due to medicine. 3. The doings of surgery are visible and manifest, while those of medicine are hidden, which is very fortunate for physicians. If they have made a mistake, it is not apparent, and if they kill the patient, it will not be done openly. But if the surgeon commits an error . . . this is seen by everybody present and cannot be attributed to nature nor to the constitution of the patient.

For hundreds of years, surgeons have been better paid than physicians. Internists will not be surprised to know how ancient is the surgeon's concern with fees. In medieval times, Mondeville was preoccupied with the matter:

The surgeon who wants to treat his patient properly must settle the matter of fee first of all. If he is not assured of his fee, he cannot concentrate on the case. He will examine superficially, and will find excuses and delays, but if he has received his fee, things are different. . . . The surgeon must have five things in mind: first, his fee; second, to avoid gossip; third, to operate cautiously; fourth, the malady; fifth, the strength of the sick man. The surgeon must not be fooled by external appearance. Wealthy people when they go to see a surgeon dress in poor clothes, or, if they are richly dressed, will tell stories in order to reduce the surgeon's salary. . . .

I have never found a man rich enough, or rather, honest enough to pay what he promised without being compelled to do so.

On the other hand, enthusiasm for operation is not an ancient vice of surgery, but a quite modern one. It was heralded by the development of anesthesia and antisepsis, both less than one hundred fifty years old. Operative restraint is still newer, a consequence of quality-control checks that are less than forty years old.

Mr. O'Connor was in the hands of the surgeons for two weeks. He was not operated upon; there was insufficient evidence of surgically treatable disease and therefore he received essentially medical treatment on the surgical wards. This is a far cry from the days when an MGH surgical chief resident told his staff (perhaps apocryphally): "Every person has at least three surgical diseases. All you have to do is find them." And it is a far cry from the days when the medical residents could accurately claim that surgeons didn't know how to read an electrocardiogram—and furthermore didn't care. In fact, there is a great deal of evidence that surgery and internal medicine are merging. It is a process that has taken several centuries, but today the cardiologists and cardiac surgeons work hand in hand, as do the immunologists and transplant surgeons; the tumor chemotherapists and the tumor surgeons; one need only look at the number of surgical house officers at the MGH who have done basic research in biochemistry and molecular biology to recognize the trend.

Bertrand Russell once said that we describe the world in mathematical terms because we are not clever enough to describe it in any more profound way. Similarly, surgeons and internists have come to see that surgery and medicine have the common goal of altering the functional status of tissues within the body. However, altering tissues with a knife is a relatively crude way of going about things; the finest surgeons are always the most reluctant to operate.

This is not to say that the scalpel will become a museum piece in our lifetime. Far from it. As surgery moves from a business of excision to a business of repair and implantation, it will be ever more important to the conduct of medicine. But the trend toward cooperation with internists, rather than competition with them, is likely to be extended as time goes on.

Indeed, the dramatics of the operating room have obscured the fact that most of the advances in surgery have taken place in terms of pre-operative and post-operative care. Modern surgery is immensely more complex than it was a century ago, but this complexity has more to do with electrolyte balances than with ligature points.

✠

One can argue that in the last twenty years surgical advance has been largely dependent on parasurgical innovation, more involved with what goes on outside the operating room than with what goes on inside it. The paradoxical effect of this has been to increase the range and variety of services directed toward the operating rooms. Vast areas of the hospital are now given over to support and maintenance of a heavy surgical schedule, involving more than 16,000 operations a year. Two clear examples are Central Supply and the Blood Bank.

"Central Supply" consists of a single large room located one floor above the operating rooms. As its name implies, it serves as the central supply room for the hundreds of sterilized articles required for the operating rooms, as well as the other floors, of the hospital. All sterilization is done here; forty-three people are employed to keep the room in operation around the clock, seven days a week. Its operating budget is more than $600,000 a year.

Excluding operating instruments, Central Supply stocks nearly 500 separate items. These include 44 kinds of Foley catheters, 29 kinds of drains, 10 kinds of needles, 15 kinds of sponges, and 55 kinds of "sets"—prepackaged collections of equipment used in carrying out special procedures. They range from alcohol nerve-block sets to arterial-oxygen sets to liver-biopsy sets to suture sets and venous-pressure sets. Each set is handed out, used, returned for re-sterilization and repackaging, and handed out again.

Altogether, Central Supply hands out 12,000 items a day, or nearly 4.5 million items a year. The work of Central Supply has been increasing markedly in recent years. For example:

HOSPITAL USE	1966	1968
Dressing sets	27,000	38,000
Suture sets	37,000	61,000
Thermometers	485,000	1,208,000

These are real figures, in the sense that they do not represent absorption of work previously done by some other area in the last two years, but rather a simple increased demand by the hospital for these items.

It should be stated at once that Central Supply does not handle all the items now required by medical technology. For instance, the ten kinds of needles it carries do not include needles for routine intramuscular and intravenous use; these are purchased presterilized and are thrown away after use. Rather, Central Supply stocks intracardiac needles, spinal needles, sternal puncture needles, ventricular needles, and other similarly specialized nondisposable apparatus.

The question of whether Central Supply should be doing as much as it does is the subject of debate. The cost of everything used in the hospital has grown so enormously that even the simplest details of patient care have undergone renewed scrutiny—revealing them, suddenly, as not so simple. Consider the Great Thermometer Controversy.

Thermometers were first used clinically in 1890, when they were delicate gadgets a foot long, but they are now a staple of modern care, and the largest item of business for Central Supply, which hands out between 3,000 and 4,000 thermometers a day. The MGH employs a method of reprocessing thermometers—unclean thermometers are returned to Central Supply, washed, sterilized, spun dry, and repackaged for use again.

The hospital recently commissioned a cost analysis of thermometer systems, which concluded that the average patient had 2.5 thermometer readings a day, and a total of 32 readings during an average admission of 13 days. Within this framework, three possible systems were examined: the reusable thermometer; a disposable probe used in conjunction with a portable sensing unit; and a personal-thermometer system in which each patient is given his own thermometer at admission, and keeps it at his bedside throughout his stay.

The conclusions on cost per year were as follows:

Reprocessable, reusable	$30,113.00
Probe and sensing unit	$49,786.00
Personal thermometer	$13,250.00

This does not tell the full story, however. There are some complicating factors. First, the present MGH system is inefficient. Central Supply does not get back all the thermometers it gives out; in 1968, it spent $30,000 to replace lost thermometers, thus effectively doubling the cost of the present system. Second, the probe and sensing unit has an important front-end cost, namely the sensing units, which cost $190 each. Amortization has not been figured into the above accounting. Neither has nursing time been assessed—and the sensing units, unlike regular thermometers, are virtually instantaneous.

The situation is further confused by fear that a personal-thermometer system may not provide adequate patient safeguards. Some have envisioned a situation in which a tuberculous patient is moved to a different room, and a new patient put in his place, with the thermometer inadvertently remaining at his bedside, to be popped into the mouth of the unsuspecting new admission. The example is farfetched, but certainly any new system deserves close scrutiny to assess its reliability and safety.

The upshot of all this is that it is difficult to be certain what is the best, safest, and cheapest way to take a patient's temperature. The problems in determining cost for this relatively simple matter are magnified many times when one attempts to unravel the cost of a radiological unit or a chemistry laboratory. Given the vagaries of accounting methods, and the uncertainty of reliability with different systems, it becomes extraordinarily difficult to decide which costs are justified and which are not.

The controversy rages on, but on balance the cost advantages are too great, and the potential for danger too little, to permit the hospital to disregard the personal-thermometer system. Converting to this system would save the hospital only five hundredths of one per cent of its annual budget. But one can see how a series of similar minor cost changes could ultimately affect total hospitalization cost.

The Blood Bank is another large and expensive facility. The MGH now has what is believed to be the largest single hospital blood bank and transfusion service in the world. Located on two floors of the Gray Building, it accounts for one fifth of all the blood used in the state of Massachusetts. The great majority of the blood goes to surgical patients, with a large proportion going to open-heart cases. At times as much as a third of all hospital blood has gone to the cardiac surgical service. This massive consumption, in turn, is largely the consequence of the heart-lung machines, which require large amounts of blood to "prime" the pump.

Although the size of the Blood Bank is closely related to the increasing demand of cardiac surgery, its growth preceded the development of open-heart techniques. The MGH Blood Bank was begun in 1942, under the part-time direction of Dr. Lamar Soutter. The hospital, skeptical of the need for such a thing, contributed $5,000 in equipment and a basement room in one of the buildings. Soutter recalls that "in the beginning everything went wrong [but] the effort paid off with unexpected rapidity. In November of 1942 the Hospital was flooded with victims of the Cocoanut Grove [fire] disaster. The Bank had more than enough plasma to give the patients adequate care. This single episode swept away the last of the opposition to the Bank and it became firmly established as a necessary part of the Hospital."

The Bank has always operated in the black, though its operating budget has grown from $5,000 in 1942 to $144,000 in 1951, and finally to more than $1 million yearly at the present time. The staff has grown from one nurse, one technician, a part-time maid, and a part-time physician in 1942 to more than one hundred technicians and nurses and secretaries at present.

✠

By definition, an organ is a mass of specialized cells serving some specific function. According to this definition, blood is an organ, though one does not often think of it in this way.

As a developing organ in the embryo, blood is formed from the same tissue which also differentiates into cartilage, connective tissue, and bone. This helps explain why, for example, blood is formed in bone marrow.

In the adult man, blood consists of five quarts of liquid, accounting for 7 per cent of adult body weight. This makes it, on a weight basis, a respectably large organ—much larger than either the lungs (1 per cent) or the liver (2 per cent). The functions of blood are suitably complex, ranging from transport of oxygen and nutrients to defense of the body against infection.

If blood is an organ, a blood transfusion is an organ

transplantation. It is not idle to think of transfusions in this way, for nearly all the problems of modern organ transplantation were first met, and solved, in dealing with blood transfusion. Only our familiarity with modern transfusion makes us forget that it is, in fact, a transplant—a gift of vital cells from donor to recipient.

No one knows when the first transfusion was performed, but it was certainly a long time ago, for the efficacy of blood was highly regarded in ancient times. In early accounts, it is not clear whether the blood was transfused or drunk, since both methods were considered useful. Celsus, in Roman times, refers to treatment of epilepsy by drinking the hot blood from the cut throat of a gladiator. The Mongols, living in a horse culture, often drank horse blood for sustenance.

The idea of intravenous injection is also old. Ovid relates that Jason was helped by Medea with an injection of "succis" into his jugular vein.

Behind the early interest in transfusion was the quite logical notion that an illness involving blood loss was best treated with blood replacement. Early materials for this were primitive—needles made of quills and bone, tubing formed from bladders or leather. In many cases, animal blood was transfused to human beings, often with the addition of semen, urine, and other substances thought to be invigorating.

It is not surprising that patients often died from this procedure. Donors often died, as well. In a famous instance, Pope Innocent VIII received a transfusion from three young boys in 1492. The donors as well as the recipient expired within a few days.

In the eighteenth century, when better materials were available and more careful observation the rule, it became clear that certain patients benefited from transfusion but others did not. This early notion of the "transfusion reaction" evolved slowly, culminating in Karl Landsteiner's discovery in 1900 of A, B, and O blood groups. This represented the first clear, unequivocal statement that all blood was not the same. For more than a decade after Landsteiner's work, there was no practical clinical method of differentiating blood groups. The search for such techniques is a direct forerunner of modern tissue-typing methods for transplantation of other organs.

Just as the matching of donor and recipient was a problem, so was storage of the organ. Untreated, blood clots soon after it is drawn. It was not until 1916 that blood could be kept refrigerated for two weeks in glass bottles, with the addition of anti-coagulating substances. And it was not for more than twenty years after that that clinical blood banking began on any scale in this country. There was no important improvement in storage techniques until 1952, when glass bottles were replaced by plastic bags, which preserved blood elements much better.

More recently has come the ability to store frozen blood. This single technical capability has solved several traditional banking problems, and indeed is now integral to the MGH function: most open-heart cases are done with frozen blood.*

Formerly, all blood had to be used within three weeks. Now it can be stored at −120°F. for five years or more. In the past, patients had to be matched to their own blood type. Now, the freezing-thawing process washes out serum antibodies, which means that type O frozen blood can be transfused to anyone, regardless of his blood type. The need for the bank to stock many different blood types is therefore reduced.

And, finally, there is evidence that the risk of hepatitis, a traditional problem with transfusions, is reduced when frozen blood is used.

There are, of course, some drawbacks to frozen blood. It is more expensive at the present time. Also, some blood components, notably platelets, which are important to clotting, are lost and must be supplied separately. But there are easy techniques for this.

In fact, the products of the modern blood bank are increasingly sophisticated. In 1942, the bank produced only two products—whole blood and plasma (the liquid portion without the cells). But it is now possible to give whole blood, or packed red cells without plasma, or platelets; it is possible to give plasma, or only the protein from the plasma, or only specific parts of the total protein without the others. Each of these specialized

* Dr. Charles Huggins, an MGH surgeon, was one of the pioneers in making frozen blood practical for clinical use.

blood bank products is becoming increasingly important to the conduct of modern medicine.

✠

What has all this meant to surgery? As it has become more scientific and more complex, a certain amount of the drama and flair, the spectacle that Warren remembered, has disappeared—or at least become muted, until it is hardly recognizable.

On Saturday mornings at the hospital, surgical clinics are held for students in which patients are presented preoperatively and then the students are invited to watch the procedures from the several overhead viewing galleries. This teaching exercise is the last remnant of a proud tradition of surgical spectacle. Dr. E. D. Churchill, former MGH Chief of Surgery, gives the following account:

The display of operations at the Hospital on Saturday mornings continued well into the 1920's. Unusual cases were assembled so that the senior surgeons on duty could have an impressive list of operations scheduled for the amphitheater. The two services, East and West, vied with each other in trying to stage the better show. In the Surgical Building, opened in 1900, the display reached major proportions. When the morning's list was a long one, an operation would be started in a small room and then the entire outfit trundled like a troupe of gypsies into the pit of the amphitheater, where the crucial phase of the procedure was demonstrated to the visiting doctors. The surgeons would be allotted, say, fifteen minutes. Whether or not the operation had been completed, at the expiration of the allotted time the tents were folded, the troupe moved off stage to complete the operation elsewhere, and a new act took over. . . . Great weight was placed on the speed and daring of the operator. . . . Tension mounted when some prima donna showed reluctance to withdraw from the spotlight and overstayed his time to hold the audience spellbound in an ad lib recounting of his surgical prowess.

The prowess of the surgeon has steadily increased since then, to the point where reconstructing a nearly severed hand is, if not commonplace, at least nothing to get very excited about.

And if, in this age of television, the surgeon shows more flamboyance than is scientifically necessary, more sense of drama than is medically indicated, he can at least be excused for upholding the traditions of his calling—and, in a deeper sense, the facts of his life.

SYLVIA THOMPSON

MEDICAL TRANSITION

Flight 404 from Los Angeles to Boston was somewhere over eastern Ohio when Mrs. Sylvia Thompson, a fifty-six-year-old mother of three, began to experience chest pain.

The pain was not severe, but it was persistent. After the aircraft landed, she asked an airline official if there was a doctor at the airport. He directed her to the Logan Airport Medical Station, at Gate 23, near the Eastern Airlines terminal.

Entering the waiting area, Mrs. Thompson told the secretary that she would like to see a doctor.

"Are you a passenger?" the secretary said.

"Yes," Mrs. Thompson said.

"What seems to be the matter?"

"I have a pain in my chest."

"The doctor will see you in just a minute," the secretary said. "Please take a seat."

Mrs. Thompson sat down. From her chair, she could look across the reception area to the computer console behind the secretary, and beyond to the small pharmacy and dispensary of the station. She could see three of the six nurses who run the station around the clock. It was now two in the afternoon, and the station was relatively quiet; earlier in the day a half dozen people had come in for yellow fever vaccinations, which are given every Tuesday and Saturday morning. But now the only other patient she could see was a young airplane mechanic who had cut his finger and was having it cleaned in the treatment room down the corridor.

A nurse came over and checked her blood pressure, pulse, and temperature, writing the information down on a slip of paper.

The door to the room nearest Mrs. Thompson was closed. From inside, she heard muffled voices. After several minutes, a stewardess came out and closed the door behind her. The stewardess arranged her next appointment with the secretary, and left.

The secretary turned to Mrs. Thompson. "The doctor will talk with you now," she said, and led Mrs. Thompson into the room that the stewardess had just left.

It was pleasantly furnished with drapes and a carpet.

There was an examining table and a chair; both faced a television console. Beneath the TV screen was a remote-control television camera. Over in another corner of the room was a portable camera on a rolling tripod. In still another corner, near the examining couch, was a large instrument console with gauges and dials.

"You'll be speaking with Dr. Murphy," the secretary said.

A nurse then came into the room and motioned Mrs. Thompson to take a seat. Mrs. Thompson looked uncertainly at all the equipment. On the screen, Dr. Raymond Murphy was looking down at some papers on his desk.

The nurse said: "Dr. Murphy."

Dr. Murphy looked up. The television camera beneath the TV screen made a grinding noise, and pivoted around to train on the nurse.

"Yes?"

"This is Mrs. Thompson from Los Angeles. She is a passenger, fifty-six years old, and she has chest pain. Her blood pressure is 120/80, her pulse is 78, and her temperature is 101.4."

Dr. Murphy nodded. "How do you do, Mrs. Thompson."

Mrs. Thompson was slightly flustered. She turned to the nurse. "What do I do?"

"Just talk to him. He can see you through that camera there, and hear you through that microphone." She pointed to the microphone suspended from the ceiling.

"But where is he?"

"I'm at the Massachusetts General Hospital," Dr. Murphy said. "When did you first get this pain?"

"Today, about two hours ago."

"In flight?"

"Yes."

"What were you doing when it began?"

"Eating lunch. It's continued since then."

"Can you describe it for me?"

"It's not very strong, but it's sharp. In the left side of my chest. Over here," she said, pointing. Then she caught herself, and looked questioningly at the nurse.

"I see," Dr. Murphy said. "Does the pain go anywhere? Does it move around?"

"No."

"Do you have pain in your stomach, or in your teeth, or in either of your arms?"

"No."

"Does anything make it worse or better?"

"It hurts when I take a deep breath."

"Have you ever had it before?"

"No. This is the first time."

"Have you ever had any trouble with your heart or lungs before?"

She said she had not. The interview continued for several minutes more, while Dr. Murphy determined that she had no striking symptoms of cardiac disease, that she smoked a pack of cigarettes a day, and that she had a chronic unproductive cough.

He then said, "I'd like you to sit on the couch, please. The nurse will help you disrobe."

Mrs. Thompson moved from the chair to the couch. The remote-control camera whirred mechanically as it followed her. The nurse helped Mrs. Thompson undress. Then Dr. Murphy said: "Would you point to where the pain is, please?"

Mrs. Thompson pointed to the lower-left chest wall, her finger describing an arc along the ribs.

"All right. I'm going to listen to your lungs and heart now."

The nurse stepped to the large instrument console and began flicking switches. She then applied a small, round metal stethoscope to Mrs. Thompson's chest. On the TV screen, Mrs. Thompson saw Dr. Murphy place a stethoscope in his ears.

"Just breathe easily with your mouth open," Dr. Murphy said.

For some minutes he listened to breath sounds, directing the nurse where to move the stethoscope. He then asked Mrs. Thompson to say "ninety-nine" over and over, while the stethoscope was moved. At length he shifted his attention to the heart.

"Now I'd like you to lie down on the couch," Dr. Murphy said, and directed that the stethoscope be removed. To the nurse: "Put the remote camera on Mrs. Thompson's face. Use a close-up lens."

"An eleven hundred?" the nurse asked.

"An eleven hundred will be fine."

The nurse wheeled the remote camera over from the corner of the room and trained it on Mrs. Thompson's face. In the meantime, Dr. Murphy adjusted his own camera so that it was looking at her abdomen.

"Mrs. Thompson," Dr. Murphy said, "I'll be watching both your face and your stomach as the nurse palpates your abdomen. Just relax now."

He then directed the nurse, who felt different areas of the abdomen. None was tender.

"I'd like to look at the feet now," Dr. Murphy said. With the help of the nurse, he checked them for edema. Then he looked at the neck veins.

"Mrs. Thompson, we're going to take a cardiogram now."

The proper leads were attached to the patient. On the TV screen, she watched Dr. Murphy turn to one side and look at a thin strip of paper.

The nurse said: "The cardiogram is transmitted directly to him."

"Oh my," Mrs. Thompson said. "How far away is he?"

"Two and a half miles," Dr. Murphy said, not looking up from the cardiogram.

✠

While the examination was proceeding, another nurse was preparing samples of Mrs. Thompson's blood and urine in a laboratory down the hall. She placed the samples under a microscope attached to a TV camera. Watching on a monitor, she could see the image that was being transmitted to Dr. Murphy. She could also talk directly with him, moving the slide about as he instructed.

Mrs. Thompson had a white count of 18,000. Dr. Murphy could clearly see an increase in the different kinds of white cells. He could also see that the urine was clean, with no evidence of infection.

Back in the examining room, Dr. Murphy said: "Mrs. Thompson, it looks like you have a pneumonia. We'd like you to come into the hospital for X rays and further evaluation. I'm going to give you something to make you a little more comfortable."

He directed the nurse to write a prescription. She then carried it over to the telewriter, above the equipment console. Using the telewriter unit at the MGH, Dr. Murphy signed the prescription.

Afterward, Mrs. Thompson said: "My goodness. It was just like the real thing."

❖

When she had gone, Dr. Murphy discussed both her case and the television link-up.

"We think it's an interesting system," he said, "and it has a lot of potential. It's interesting that patients accept it quite well. Mrs. Thompson was a little hesitant at first, but very rapidly became accustomed to the system. There's a reason—talking by closed-circuit TV is really very little different from direct, personal interviews. I can see your facial expression, and you can see mine; we can talk to each other quite naturally. It's true that we are both in black and white, not color, but that's not really important. It isn't even important for dermatologic diagnoses. You might think that color would be terribly important in examining a skin rash, but it's not. The history a patient gives and the distribution of the lesions on the body and their shape give important clues. We've had very good success diagnosing rashes in black and white, but we do need to evaluate this further.

"The system we have here is pretty refined. We can look closely at various parts of the body, using different lenses and lights. We can see down the throat; we can get close enough to examine pupillary dilation. We can easily see the veins on the whites of the eyes. So it's quite adequate for most things.

"There are some limitations, of course. You have to instruct the nurse in what to do, in your behalf. It takes time to arrange the patient, the cameras, and the lighting, to make certain observations. And for some procedures, such as palpating the abdomen, you have to rely heavily on the nurse, though we can watch for muscle spasm and facial reaction to pain—that kind of thing.

"We don't claim that this is a perfect system by any

126

means. But it's an interesting way to provide a doctor to an area that might not otherwise have one."

✠

Boston's Logan Airport is the eighth busiest in the world. In addition to the steady stream of incoming and outgoing passengers, there are more than 5,000 airport employees. The problem of providing medical care to this population has been a difficult one for many years. Like many populations, it is too large to be ignored, but too small to support a full-time physician in residence. Nor can a physician easily make the journey back and forth from the hospital to the airport; though only 2.7 miles away, the airport is, practically speaking, isolated for many hours of the day by rush-hour traffic congestion.

The solution of Dr. Kenneth T. Bird, who runs the unit, has been to provide a physician when the patient demand is heaviest, and to provide additional coverage by television. The system now used, called Tele-Diagnosis, is frankly experimental. It has been in operation for slightly more than a year. At the present time, eight to ten patients a day are interviewed and examined by television.

The Logan TV system is probably the first of its kind in the country, but Bird refuses to discuss priority. "The first to have it," he says, "was Tom Swift, in 1914."

Certainly there is a science-fiction quality about the

station's equipment, for along with the Tele-Diagnosis apparatus, there is also a time-sharing station linked to the hospital's computer. Among other things, this computer can be used to take a preliminary history—to function as a doctor in questioning the patient about his symptoms and their nature. Some 15 per cent of the patients examined by Tele-Diagnosis have had their medical history taken by computer before they see the doctor himself. Like the cardiogram, the computer history can be sent directly to the physician.

Being interviewed by a machine is less bizarre than it sounds. Indeed, like the TV link-up, it is remarkable for the ease with which patients accept it. The most common complaint is boredom: the machine sometimes pauses three or four seconds between questions, and the patients get fidgety.

To be interviewed, one sits in front of a teletype console. The computer asks questions, which are printed out, and the patient punches in his answers. Whenever the computer gets a "yes" answer to some question, it follows it up with more questions on the same subject. If it gets a "no" answer, it goes on to the next topic. At the conclusion of the question, the computer writes out a medical summary. Unlike the questions, the summary is phrased in medical terminology. The entire process takes roughly half an hour.

The result of one such interview is reprinted in part below. The computer was given the same presenting complaint as that of Mrs. Thompson: chest pain. In an attempt to confuse it, the machine was first fed some false but suggestive information, namely, that there was a family history of cardiovascular disease, and that the patient was taking digitalis. However, in later questions, the machine was given a straightforward history for the type of chest pain most common among medical students—that of psychogenic, or musculoskeletal, origin.

A sample of the questions and answers ran as follows:

68 HAS YOUR VOICE CHANGED(BECOME ROUGH, SCRATCHY OR HOARSE) DURING THE PAST YEAR?

■9 NO

69 DO YOU HAVE A COUGH?

■8 YES

70 HOW LONG HAVE YOU HAD THE COUGH?
1, A FEW DAYS
2, A FEW WEEKS
3, SEVERAL MONTHS
4, A FEW YEARS

■3

67 DO YOU HAVE THIS COUGH EVERY DAY?

■8 YES

71 DO YOU BRING UP ANY MATERIAL(SUCH AS SPUTUM, PHLEGM, OR MUCUS) FROM YOUR CHEST?

■9 NO

74 HAVE YOU EVER COUGHED UP BLOOD?

■9 NO

At the conclusion of these and other questions, the computer printed the following summary:

MEDICAL HISTORY SUMMARY   DATE: MAY 27, 1969

NAME: MICHAEL CRICHTON   UNIT#: DEMO

AGE: 26   SEX: MALE

CHIEF COMPLAINT: CHEST PAIN

COMMUNITY PHYSICIAN: NONE

OCCUPATION: MEDICAL STUDENT

MEDICATIONS: DIGITALIS

DRUG REACTIONS: PAN ALBA

HOSPITALIZATIONS: NONE

FAMILY HISTORY: HEART ATTACK, HYPERTENSION.

SOCIAL HISTORY
   PT. IS MARRIED, HAS NO CHILDREN. COLLEGE GRADUATE.
PRESENTLY A STUDENT, WORKING 50-60 HRS/WK. HAS BEEN
SMOKING 5-10 YRS, 1 PACK/DAY. ALCOHOLIC CONSUMPTION:
1 DRINK/DAY. FOREIGN TRAVEL WITHIN THE LAST 10 YEARS.

REVIEW OF SYSTEMS

GENERAL HEALTH
   NO SIGNIFICANT WEIGHT CHANGE IN PAST YEAR. SLEEPS
6-8 HRS/NIGHT. HEAD INJURIES: NONE WITHIN PAST 5 YRS.
EYE SYMPTOMS: NONE. HAS BEEN TOLD BY MD OF NO EYE
DISEASE. NO TINNITUS. NO EPISTAXIS, NOTES SINUS
TROUBLE. DENIES CHANGE IN VOICE.

RESPIRATORY SYSTEM
   PT. NOTES COUGH OF SEVERAL MONTHS DURATION, WHICH
OCCURS DAILY. DENIES SPUTUM PRODUCTION, DENIES
HEMOPTYSIS. NOTES NO DYSPNEA. HAS HAD HAY FEVER.
HAS HAD NO KNOWN CONTACT WITH TUBERCULOSIS. LAST
CHEST X-RAY 12 YRS AGO.

CARDIOVASCULAR SYSTEM
PT. NOTES CHEST PAIN OCCURRING LESS THAN ONCE A
MONTH, LOCATED "ON BOTH SIDES", WHICH RADIATES TO
NEITHER ARM NOR NECK. PAIN IS NOT AFFECTED BY DEEP
BREATHING, IS NOT ASSOCIATED WITH EATING, EMOTION,
OR EXERCISE. PAIN IS NOT RELIEVED BY RESTING.
PT. NOTES PALPITATIONS ON RARE OCCASIONS. DENIES
ORTHOPNEA. DENIES PEDAL EDEMA. DENIES LEG PAINS,
DENIES VARICOSE VEINS. DENIES PERIPHERAL REACTION
TO COLD. CARDIAC MEDICATIONS: NONE. HAS BEEN TOLD
BY MD OF NO COMMON CARDIAC DISEASE. NO ECG IN PAST
2 YRS.

This is only half the total report. Analysis of gastro-intestinal musculoskeletal, genito-urinary, hematologic, endocrine, dermatologic, and neurological systems followed. This particular computer program draws no conclusions about diagnosis; it only summarizes answers to its own questions, and it does not cross-check itself. Thus, while the computer was told the patient took digitalis, it later accepted the conflicting statement that the patient took no cardiac medication.

This program, which was devised at the MGH, is a rather simple example of the way that computers can and almost certainly will be used in the future. But it is the least sophisticated of the medical-history programs available; more complex ones already exist.

✠

When Mrs. Thompson arrived at the MGH emergency ward, which had been expecting her, she was taken down to the EW X-ray department. In doing so, she passed a door near the front of the EW which is unmarked, without a label. Over the door is a lighted sign that says, incongruously, "On Air."

Dr. Murphy was behind that door, sitting in a corner of a small room, surrounded by equipment. Directly in front of him was a camera and a large TV screen, on which he watches the Logan patients. Built into his desk were two other screens: one, a small monitor of the larger screen, the other, a monitor that showed him his own image being transmitted to the patient. This second monitor allowed him to check his own facial expressions, the light in the room, and so on.

To his right was a panel of buttons that controlled the various remote cameras—two in the examining room and one in the laboratory. The examining-room remote camera is operated by a joystick: by pushing the stick right or left, up or down, the camera moves accordingly. In addition, there are buttons for focusing and zoom control.

Before going out to check on Mrs. Thompson, Dr. Murphy continued a study of Tele-Diagnosis capability: reading a series of 120 chest X rays that are set up for him at Logan. He planned to read these by TV and later reread them in person, to compare the accuracy and consistency of his diagnosis.

The nurse at Logan set up the next X ray.

"What's this one?"

"Jay-nineteen," the nurse said, reading off the code number.

"Okay." He moved the joystick and touched the buttons. The camera tracked around the X ray, examining the ribs, then scanning the lung fields. "Wait a minute." He zoomed in to look closely at the right-upper lobe; he watched the little monitor, because resolution was better, but by glancing up at the large screen, he could also get a magnified view. "No. Well, on second thought . . ." He zoomed back for an over-all view. He zoomed in on another part of the upper lobe. "Looks like a small cavitation there . . ." He zoomed back, touching the buttons. He turned to the joystick, panned across the rest of the lung field, occasionally pausing to look at suspicious areas. "Nothing else, not really . . ." He finished his scan, and returned to the right-upper lobe. "Yes, there's cavitation. I'd have to call it moderately advanced tuberculosis. Next, please."

He was working with considerable rapidity. "You get to be pretty good at this," he said. "At first, it all seems clumsy, but as you get more accustomed to the equipment, you move faster."

The average time for a patient interview and examination by Tele-Diagnosis is now twelve minutes, less than half the average figure a year ago.

"What I'm doing now," he said, "is really just a test of our capability. It has no immediate practical use, because we can't take X rays at Logan—that's one of the main reasons we brought Mrs. Thompson into the hospital. But it's important to know if X rays can be read at a distance with accuracy. Our impression is that you can read them as well on TV as you can in person.

"Jay-twenty," the nurse said, putting up another film. Murphy began his scan. "Ah. What's this? Looks like a rib fracture . . ."

✠

One can argue that for the past twenty years technology has defined the hospital, has made it what it is today. That is, once a range of expensive, complex therapeutic and diagnostic machinery became available, the hospital assumed the role of providing a central location for such equipment. This was inevitable: private practitioners and even large group practices could not afford to buy such equipment, nor maintain it, nor pay the personnel to operate it. Only the hospital could do this. It was the only institution in existence that could possibly absorb the expense. Other possible institutions, such as nursing homes, were wholly inadequate.

Furthermore, because the hospital was already oriented toward acute care of critically ill patients, the technology that it absorbed was precisely that which helped in this area. Monitoring machines and life-support equipment are clear examples. Thus technology reinforced an already existing trend.

Now, however, the pressures and forces acting upon the hospital are social and of a nature that is changing the meaning of technology within the hospital. As C. P. Snow has said, "We have been letting technology run us as if we had no judgment of our own." But such judg-

134

ment is now required, and one can argue that in the next twenty years the hospital will define technology. That is, it will create a demand for new technological applications—and in certain ways will itself produce the new technology.

By doing this, the hospital will be extending its newest and most striking trend, which is to foster innovation, later to be picked up by other, nonacademic institutions. The absurd end-point of such a trend would be for the hospital to direct personally the diagnosis and therapy of a patient who never entered the hospital. Absurd as it may be, it is already happening in the case of many patients treated at Logan Airport. It will happen more often, in other ways, in the future.

Of the almost limitless spectrum of potential technological advance, we can concentrate here on two areas of imminent advance, television and computers. One ought to say that they have been imminent for a long time; a decade ago one heard that computers were about to revolutionize medicine, and one still hears it today. It obviously hasn't happened yet. Indeed, neither television nor the computer has made much difference yet to routine hospital functioning. Television is employed on occasion for student teaching; it is used in a small way for dispatching blood samples and other items; it has some application in X-ray technology, in terms of image-intensification systems. Computers remain primarily the plaything of researchers. At the MGH there is now a computer program to help in running the clinical chemistry lab, and a computer to help in billing and patient record-keeping, but the computer and television as direct aids in patient care have not made their appearance.

In contrast, the Tele-Diagnosis system at Logan Airport uses computers and TV in direct confrontation with the patient. The system is expensive and in some ways primitive. Also, its present thrust is diagnostic; therapy, the steps following diagnosis, will still be directly carried out by a doctor, nurse, or the patient himself. There are no machines to do this, unless one stretches the definition to include renal-dialysis machines, exercise machines, and the like.

In general, diagnostic automation appears much closer than therapeutic automation—and is much more readily acceptable to physicians. Consider, then, diagnostic automation first.

The first and most striking feature of the Logan system is that diagnosis can occur at a distance. The doctor's stethoscope is three miles long. But, oddly, that is the least original aspect of the situation. In medicine, diagnosis at a distance is very old and has some humorous elements. Beginning around A.D. 900, for example, the practice of uroscopy, or "water casting," came into vogue. It was felt that the amount of information obtainable from inspection of urine was unlimited. The urine of a sick man was often sent many miles to be examined by a prominent physician.

David Riesman cites a typical medieval interpretation of urine:

The urine is pale pink, thick above, thin below, becoming gray or dark toward the surface. The grayness and obscurity is caused by overheating of the material. The symptoms are these: pain in the head, especially in the temples, sourness of the breath, pains in the back from bile descending to the loins and kidneys, with paroxysms every day or every second day, usually coming on after dinner time.

In medieval literature there are many discussions of the hazards to the physician of uroscopy; even in those days, diagnosis at a distance had its risks. The Spanish physician Arnold of Villanova, who lived in the thirteenth century, wrote:

With regard to urines, we must consider the precautions to protect ourselves against people who wish to deceive us. The very first shall consist in finding out whether the urine be of man or of another animal or another fluid.

The second precaution is with regard to the individual who brings the urine. You must look at him sharply and keep your eyes straight on him or on his face; and if he wishes to deceive you he will start laughing, or the color of his face will change, and then you must curse him forever and in all eternity.

The third precaution is also with regard to the individual who brings the urine, whether man or woman, for you must see whether he or she is pale, and after you have ascertained that this is the individual's urine, say to him: "Verily, this urine resembles you," and talk about the pallor, because immediately you will hear all about his illness. . . .

The fourth precaution is with regard to sex. An old woman wants to have your opinion. You inquire whose urine it is, and the old woman will say to you: "Don't you know it?" Then look at her in a certain way from the corner of your eye, and ask: "What relation is it of yours?" And if she is not too crooked, she will say that the patient is a male or female relation, or something from which you can distinguish the sex. . . . Or ask what the patient used to do when he was in good health, and from the patient's doing you can recognize or deduce the sex. . . .

The list continues through nineteen precautions, all designed to enable the physician to pry information from the person bringing the urine, and to prevent deception. Arnold was not above a little deception himself, however:

You may not find anything about the case. Then say that he has an obstruction of the liver, and particularly use the word, obstruction, because they do not understand what it means, and it helps greatly that a term is not understood by the people.

The modern counterpart of this medieval guessing game over urine is the telephone conversation between physician and patient. For years after the telephone became common, physicians resisted making telephone diagnoses, and they still frown on them. But every practicing doctor now spends a substantial part of his day

138

talking to patients on the phone, and he is resigned to making a large number of decisions, some of them uneasily, by phone.

Closed-circuit television, while far from the ideal of a personal examination, is vastly superior to the telephone alone, and in many cases it is surprisingly adequate. This does not mean that future patients will all be seen by closed-circuit television, with neither doctor nor patient leaving home. What it does mean is that television will probably work in certain very special applications. One of these is the Logan application—providing a doctor to a clinic during low-use periods. Another obvious use would be specialist consultations. A hospital or clinic that needs a neurologist only a few times a year cannot afford to staff one. Nor could it find one, even if it could afford it. Television is perfectly suited to such consultation.

At the same time, a system such as that at Logan makes possible a routine physical examination, but goes no further—and there are suggestions that technology will ultimately change the very nature of physical examination. Here the historical trend is clear.

Consider the innovations in physical diagnosis. In the nineteenth century, there were three of great importance—the stethoscope, the blood-pressure cuff, and the thermometer. Each of these is really nothing more than a precise way to determine what can be inaccurately determined by other means. Thus the thermometer is superior to the hand on the forehead; the stethoscope superior to the ear against the chest*; and the blood-pressure cuff superior to a finger compressing the artery to test its pressure.

Now, the first two advances of the twentieth century were quite different: the X ray and electrocardiogram provided new information not obtainable by physical contact. No amount of squeezing and touching the patient will tell you anything directly about the electrical currents in his heart. You may deduce this information from other findings, but you cannot extract it directly. Similarly, X rays represent a new kind of vision, providing a new kind of information.

At the present time a variety of examination procedures are being tested. These include thermography, ultraviolet light, ultrasonic sound, as well as mapping electrical currents in the skin. Except for thermography, these all represent "new" sensory information for the doctor.

Thus the initial trend was to measure the patient more exactly, and later, to measure the patient in new ways. The first approach has been to find new sorts of measurements and new sensory information. But a second approach, now in its infancy, concerns translation of old information into new forms. The computer will be helpful here in a number of ways, in producing what is called "derivative information."

* For the purposes of this argument, I will ignore the fact that the stethoscope really initiated auscultation as a useful examination procedure. In truth, ears were not pressed against the chest with much regularity before Laënnec invented the stethoscope and described auscultation.

In a simple way, this is already being done. The human computer* and the electrocardiogram are a clear example. The electrocardiogram measures electrical currents within the heart muscle—the current that makes it contract and beat. Often, when a physician looks at an electrocardiogram, he wants specific electrical information. He wants to know about rate and rhythm, about conduction of impulses, and so on. At other times, he wants non-electrical information. He may want to know how thick a part of the heart wall is, for instance. In this case, he derives the information from the electrical information.

But there are more complex forms of derived information. A physician examining a patient with heart disease may be interested in knowing the cardiac output —exactly how much blood the heart is pumping per minute. This is the product of heart rate (easily determined) and volume of blood ejected per beat (very difficult to determine). Because cardiac output is so hard to assess, it is not much used in diagnosis and therapy. However, by measuring heart rate and the shape of the arterial pulse (both easily done) a computer can calculate cardiac output and can perform these calculations continuously over a period of days, if necessary. If a physician needs to know cardiac output, he can have this information. He can have it for as long as the patient is connected to the computer.

Does the physician really need cardiac output? At the moment, he can't be sure. For centuries he's had to con-

---

* Defined as the only computer that can be produced by unskilled labor.

tent himself with other information. There is reason to believe, however, that cardiac output will be useful in a variety of ways, as will other derived information.

An interesting technological application concerns the reverse of the coin: determining which information the physician already has but does not need. This is not to say that the information is inaccurate, but only that it does not have diagnostic significance and is therefore not worth obtaining. At present, the physician naturally tries to avoid gathering useless information, but in certain circumstances he cannot perform as well as a computer. Multiple discriminant analysis is a case in point. As one observer notes, "There is a limitation on the human mind regarding the speed, accuracy, and ability to correlate and intercorrelate multiple variables with all possible outcomes and treatment consequences." There is a limitation on the computer, too. Practically speaking, there are many limitations. But in purely mathematical capability, the human mind is much inferior to the computer in multiple-discriminant analysis.

This is a function vital to diagnosis. It refers to the ability to consider a large body of facts, and on the basis of those facts to assign a patient to one diagnostic category or another on the basis of probability. Consider a simple set of categories: appendicitis versus no-appendicitis. (This is a simplification of what is, practically speaking, a larger problem in diagnostic categories, but it will serve to explain the principle.) Let us assume that a surgeon seeing a patient with pain on the right side must make only this decision. How does he make it? No single piece of information will tell him the answer (except, perhaps, the fact of a previous appendectomy). Certainly such routine data as sex, age, white count, degree of fever, duration of pain in hours will not tell him. But considered all together, they permit him to arrive at a decision.

This is all very familiar. But the point is that it is not very precise. A discriminant function can be produced that weighs each variable—age, sex, white count—on the basis of how important each variable has been in the past. Thus the discriminant function has two uses. First, it can make a diagnosis and act as a consultant to the surgeon.* Second, it can determine which variables are most significant, which account for the greatest proportion of the variance, in making a diagnosis. This can sometimes be surprising. For example, one study of women undergoing gynecologic surgery indicated that the age of the patient had great diagnostic importance, and that notation of last menstrual period, biopsy of smear, pre-operative hemoglobin, and urine-sediment study were all much less important to making a diagnosis.

These applications of the computer are designed to be diagnostic aids to the doctor, rather than a replacement. One hears, for example, that "even though com-

* Several discriminant functions have been made and shown to be as accurate as the surgeons, though interpretation is made more complex by the fact that these functions are generated from data on previously diagnosed patients.

puters can be programmed to make diagnoses, it takes the physician to perform the physical examination, and it takes the personal contact of the doctor-patient relationship to gather the information needed for the identification process."

For better or worse, this is not quite true. History-taking, long the province of the physician and a keystone to his "art," is partially amenable to automation. The Logan station utilizes a simple program, which is not so much a conversation with the computer as a quiz. But more sophisticated programs exist, and still better ones are being planned.

Some years ago, Joseph Weizenbaum of MIT designed a program to conduct psychiatric interviews. Although in some senses the program can be regarded as a "trick," it can nonetheless achieve impressive results. Dr. Andrew T. Weil has reported one interaction between the computer and a human psychiatrist as follows (the computer writes in upper-case letters; mere humans, in lower-case).

doctor, i have terrible news

YOU SAY YOU HAVE TERRIBLE NEWS

yes, there is a computer program at m.i.t. that'll ruin us

WHY DO YOU SAY THAT

i have seen it working

YOU SAY YOU HAVE SEEN IT WORKING

it's frightening—you must see it

YOU THINK I MUST SEE IT

you sound depressed to me

IN YOUR FANTASY PERHAPS WE SOUND DEPRESSED TO
EACH OTHER

yes—perhaps

I UNDERSTAND

i do too

YOU SAY YOU DO TOO

we are both in the same boat with respect to the computer

LET'S CONTINUE TO TALK ABOUT YOU—SHALL WE

you are a comfort

WHAT MAKES YOU THINK I AM A COMFORT

at a time like this you want to talk about me

WHY DO YOU THINK I WANT TO TALK ABOUT YOU

because you share my feelings about that damned computer

WHAT DOES THAT SUGGEST TO YOU

that, of course, you hate computers too

YOU THINK I HATE COMPUTERS TOO

why not, they're hardly human, are they

PERHAPS THAT'S WHAT WE ARE HERE TO FIND OUT

no computer could converse as you can, for example

OH

i can't understand how anyone could be fooled by a
    mere machine

CAN'T YOU REALLY

no, after all, there is nothing creative about a computer
    program

YOU ARE BEING NEGATIVE

i am convinced i am correct

ARE YOU WORRIED TO HAVE BEEN CONVINCED YOU ARE CORRECT

no, not in the least. not at all. not even a little

YOU ARE BEING NEGATIVE

you said you agreed with me, didn't you

IS THAT WHAT YOU HEARD ME SAY

why don't you try to dissuade me—computers diddle
    with numbers that's all

YOU WISH ME TO TRY TO DISSUADE YOU

you can't

YOU THINK I CAN'T

for example, could a computer in conversation like this raise a new topic

YOU SEEM TO HAVE AVOIDED SPEAKING OF YOUR PARENTS ALTOGETHER

precisely as you just did

YOU THINK I JUST DID

yes, and that's what shows the difference between a man and a computer

I SEE

This kind of interaction is suggestive, at least of the ways computers can be utilized in the future. And as the hospital reaches out into the community, these may be increasingly important. According to Jerome Grossman of the MGH Computer Sciences Laboratory, "A large part of history-taking is directed toward finding out how sick a person really is. The first question is always whether a patient needs to see a doctor at all. That's the biggest decision doctors make over the phone now —talking to the patients, trying to decide whether they're sick enough to be seen now, or whether it can wait. The patients want to know the same thing, so they spend all night or all weekend trying to get hold of the doctor, who's off duty, or out of town, or something. . . .

"In the near future, when the home computer and television set is practical, you're going to be able to plug right into the hospital computer without ever leaving your home. The computer will flash questions on the screen, like 'Do you have a cough?' and you answer by touching the screen with your finger at the appropriate place. We've just developed a screen like this. It doesn't require any special gadgets or light pens or anything, just your finger. Touch the screen, and the information is recorded. Eventually, the computer will flash back some directions, like 'Come to the hospital immediately' or 'Call your doctor in the morning' or 'Have a check-up within six weeks,' or 'Someone will come on the screen, if further classification is necessary.' So there you have it. That first big decision—who needs to be seen—is settled by the computer, without ever having required the doctor's presence."

The idea is interesting not because it is an imminent practical development—it is not*—but rather that it represents a further extension of the hospital into the community—not only into clinics via TV, but into the home of many individuals, via computer. One can argue, in fact, that those who predict the hospital's role as "primary physician" or "first-contact physician" is declining are wrong. It will ultimately increase with the use of computers.

---

* What *is* imminent is the use of computer stations to take a portion of routine history and to advise the doctor on further tests. Such consoles are already in use experimentally in the MGH medical clinics and in certain private doctors' offices.

148

✠

Automated diagnosis is one thing; automated therapy, quite another. It is probably fair to say it is feared equally by both patients and physicians. It is also important to state firmly that the following discussion is largely speculative; automated diagnosis is in its infancy, but automated therapy has hardly been conceived. Its modern forerunners are the monitoring systems that check vital signs and the electrocardiogram. These monitors are not computers at all, in any real sense; they are just mechanical watchdogs, about as sophisticated as a burglar alarm.

At the present time, there are serious problems facing anyone who wishes to automate the therapy of even a circumscribed class or category of patient. To automate the therapy of all patients, with the full spectrum of disease, would be an enormous undertaking. Whether or not it is done will depend largely upon the demand for it, which in turn depends upon the availability of physicians. In assuming that it will be done, at least to some extent, I have also assumed that the shortage of physicians in this country will increase in the foreseeable future, necessitating a practical change in the doctor's functions.

Partially automated therapy is already desirable. The reasons are twofold. First, modern therapy makes necessary an enormous amount of paperwork; one hospital study concluded that 25 per cent of the hospital budget was devoted to information processing. The usual hospital systems for collecting, filing, and retrieving information consume great quantities of time for nearly everyone working in the hospital, from the physician who must spend time thumbing through the chart, to the nurses who must record routine data, to the personnel who work full time in the chart-record storage rooms. One consequence of the present methods, aside from the expense, is the number of errors that occur at various points along the line. And the possible advantage of putting all data through computers is the ability to check errors. For instance, if medications are ordered by the physician through a computer, that computer can tirelessly review orders for drug incompatibilities, inappropriate dosages, and so on.

The second reason comes from experience with present monitors in intensive-care units. These monitors "watch" the patient more carefully than any group of physicians could; the patient's condition is sampled continuously, rather than just during rounds. Such monitoring has already changed many ideas about the nature of disease processes* and it has renewed consideration of therapy at intervals. For example, most drugs are now given every six hours, or every four hours, or on some other schedule. But why not continuously, in an appropriate dose? And in that case, why not have a machine that can correct therapy on the basis of changes in the patient's condition?

---

* One example: the incidence of cardiac arrythmia following myocardial infarction is now suspected to be virtually 100 per cent; it is thus an almost certain consequence of heart attack—this is useful information since the arrythmias are the most common cause of sudden early death from heart attack.

Seen in this light, automated therapy becomes a more reasonable prospect. It will require adjustment, of course, by both doctors and patients. But that adjustment will be no more severe than it will be in other sectors of society.

In the past fifty years, society has had to adapt to machines that do mechanical work—in essence, taking over functions of the musculoskeletal system. It is now quite accepted that almost nobody does anything "by hand" or "on foot," except for sport or pleasure. But what is coming is what Gerard Piel calls "the disemployment of the nervous system," in a manner comparable to the disemployment of the musculoskeletal system. Man has accepted the fact that there are machines superior to his body; he must now accept the fact that there are machines in many ways superior to his brain.

The image of the patient, lying alone in bed, surrounded by clicking, whirring, stainless steel is certainly unnerving. It is easy to agree with the doctors who fear automation as leading to depersonalized care, and the computer, as psychologist George Miller notes, as "synonymous with mechanical depersonalization." But that is probably because we are so unfamiliar with them, and, in any event, man has found ways to personalize machines in the past—the automobile is a baroque example—and there is no reason to think he cannot do it in the future.

One example of an attempt to computerize some elements of patient therapy is the computer-assisted burns treatment project being carried out, with the Shrine

Burn Institute, in Dr. G. Octo Barnett's Laboratory of
Computer Science at the MGH. The project director,
Kathleen Dwyer, notes that "there's no theoretical reason why you couldn't build a program to carry out some
functions of a doctor, at least for certain kinds of patients. But, practically speaking, it's a long way off."

In trying to find out why, precisely, it is a long way
off, one gets two kinds of answers. The first is that
nobody is really interested in working very hard, at the
moment, to duplicate a doctor on magnetic tape. The
second answer is that doctors don't know themselves
precisely how they operate; until doctors figure it out,
no one can program a machine to carry out the same
functions. The classic situation is that of the physician
who enters the room of a person with normal temperature, heart rate, blood pressure, and electrocardiogram,
takes one look at him and says: "He looks sick." How
did the physician arrive at that conclusion? If he can't
tell you the signals he used, then the programmers can't
computerize it.

This situation is often held up as a kind of limit on
the application of machines to medicine. How can one
imitate the "unconscious" or "instinctive" or "intui-
tive" or "experiential" functions of a doctor? But, in
fact, as Kirkland and others have pointed out, the argument is really more damaging to the reputations of physicians than machines. For, unless the doctor is flatly
guessing when he says, "The patient looks sick," he is
drawing a conclusion on the basis of some input, presumably visual. One need only identify that input—and

then plug it into the computer. But if the input is truly unidentifiable, one must strongly suspect that the doctor is guessing or expressing a prejudice.

In any event, there is considerable interest in knowing how a doctor decides that a patient looks sick, or looks better, for, as Dr. Jerome Grossman says: "Working with computers has made us look closely at how people think."

But at the moment computer-assisted programs are all that are being used. Dwyer's program, which will be in pilot use by the end of 1970, is specifically designed to help in a major management problem—the burned pediatric patient. These young patients require close monitoring and frequent changes in therapy. This in turn produces an enormous amount of paperwork and accumulated data that is hard for a physician to summarize in his own mind simply by reading the chart. Dwyer anticipates that a computer-assisted program would "facilitate the orderly collection and retrieval of information [and] would not only improve patient care . . . but would also lead to the development of optimal therapeutic models and a better understanding of the disease process."

The first phase of the project will be a simple book-keeping function: storing information about the patient and his treatment and displaying it on command on a teletype, or a cathode-ray tube (essentially, a TV screen), whenever the physician requests it. A hypothetical example of such a display is shown on the next page:

FLUID I-O   SMITH, JOHN
2/2/68 11.30AM   123-45-67

TIME	RINGERS	ORAL	URINE	WT(KG)	OTHER IV
TODAY **2/2/68**					
8AM	300/300	-	100/100	32	-
9AM	250/550	100/100	100/200	32.5	-
10AM	100/650	200/300	135/325	33	100B
11AM	200/850	50/350	122/447	32.5	-
FLUID TOTALS	INPUT: 1300		OUTPUT: 447		WT. CHANGE: +.5

TIME	RINGERS	ORAL	URINE	WT(KG)	OTHER IV
YESTERDAY **2/1/68**					
8AM	100/100	50/50	75/75	31	-
9AM	200/300	-/50	50/125	31	-
10AM	300/600	100/150	75/200	31.5	300P
11AM	300/900	100/250	100/300	31.7	-
12PM	200/1100	76/325	100/400	32	-
1PM	150/1250	-/325	150/550	-	-
•					
•					
•					
11PM	••••••••				
12AM	••••••••				
•					
•					
6AM	100/2500	-/700	200/1200	32	-
7AM	72/2575	50/750	100/1300	32	-
FLUID TOTALS	INPUT: 3325		OUTPUT: 1300		WT. CHANGE: +1

1/31/68	3000(200)/3200	1100	-1.5	B,P
1/30/68	3000(-)/3000	1000	-.5	-
1/29/68	4200(100)/4300	900	-1	-

Here the computer is summarizing intravenous (Ringers) and oral fluid intake, urine output, and weight change over a five-day period. This achievement will not be very exciting to anyone who has not spent half an hour going through a patient's chart attempting to extract this information—which the computer can provide in milliseconds.

But the second stage is rather different. It is called "computer-generated treatment regimen," and what it means is that the computer will itself advise future therapy, which the physician is free to accept or ignore. Another hypothetical example, for a new patient admitted to the unit:

```
ADMISSION DATE T 05/08/69    ADMISSION TIME N 11.22AM
ADMITTING DOCTOR'S INITIALS...KRD
PATIENT'S NAME...SMITH, JOHN
BIRTH DATE...4/20/65
UNIT NUMBER...1234567
   THIS UNIT NUMBER IS ALREADY ASSIGNED.  TRY AGAIN OR
   USE TEMP.
UNIT NUMBER...123456
LOCATION...SB1
WEIGHT(LB OR KG?)...20KG
HT(IN OR CM?)...110    IN/CM?  CM
BURN DATE T    TIME 8AM
TOTAL PERCENT BURN...36
PERCENT 1ST DEGREE...0    2ND DEGREE...9
   2ND-3RD DEGREE...27
BURN SURFACE COMPUTED TO BE 0.27 SQ. METERS
TREATED PREVIOUS TO EW
   NO
EW THERAPY
   YES    ENTER TOTALS(ML)
LAC RINGERS...200    N/S...0    PLASMA...0    BLOOD...0
URINE...0    VOMITUS...0
```

```
SUGGESTED INITIAL REPAIR AND MAINTENANCE
  1440 ML RINGERS BEFORE 4.00 PM 05/08/69
  RATE: 315 D/M PED (80 AD)
  1640 ML RINGERS BEFORE 8.00 AM 05/09/69
  RATE: 100 D/M PED


SUGGESTED INITIAL REPAIR AND MAINTENANCE
  1440 ML RINGERS BEFORE 4.00 PM AT A RATE
  OF 310 D/M (PED)
  1640 ML RINGERS BEFORE 8.00 AM ON 05/09/69 AT A RATE
  OF 100 D/M (PED)
```

Now this is not really so ominous. The suggestions for therapy are actually based on principles that come from John Crawford, chief of pediatrics at the Burns Unit. In essence, they represent (assuming no error in the program, and no variables that he would take into account but the machine does not) his therapeutic program were he personally treating the patient.

Thus the computer is at best as clever as a single clever man, and at worst considerably less astute than that one man.

Once in use, the MGH burns project will be analyzed by doctors, and adjustments made to refine the program. And as the program improves, it may become more and more difficult for a physician to ignore the computer's "advice."

In the future, it may be possible to have a computer monitor the patient and carry out therapy, maintaining the patient within certain limits established by physicians—or even by the computer itself.

The major consequence, indeed the avowed aim, of

computer therapy in any form will be to reduce the routine work of patient care done by doctors. Other elements of that care are already disappearing; nurses have taken over several of these, and technicians have taken over others. Thus, during the week, the MGH has routine blood samples drawn by technicians and routine intravenous maintenance—starting IV lines and keeping them running—done by specially trained IV nurses. These programs were quite radical a few years ago, when doctors thought nurses constitutionally incapable of dealing with intravenous lines or drawing blood from a vein. But a startling consequence of this new specialization of nonphysician health personnel has been better care, in certain areas, than the physician himself could deliver. Even if doctors don't believe this, the patients know it well. On weekends, when the IV nurses and the blood technicians are off duty, the patients complain bitterly that the physicians are not as skilled in these tasks.

As for the special skills still reserved to physicians, such as lumbar punctures and thoracic and abdominal taps, it is only a matter of time before someone discovers that these, too, can be effectively delegated to other personnel.

It would thus appear that all the functions of a doctor are being taken over either by other people or by machines. What will be left to the doctor of the future?

Almost certainly he will begin to move in one of two directions. The first is clearly toward full-time research.

The last fifteen years have seen a striking increase in the number of hospital-based physicians and the number of doctors conducting research in governmental agencies. This trend will almost surely continue.

A second direction will be away from science toward the "art" of medicine—the complex, very human problems of helping people adjust to disease processes; for there will always be a gap between the illnesses medicine faces and science's limitations in treating them. And there will always be a need for people to bridge that gap.

Physicians moving in either direction will be helped by a new freedom from the details of patient care; and physicians now emotionally attached to those details, such as those doctors who religiously insist on doing their own lab work, are mistaking the nature of their trade. Almost invariably, they would do better spending their time talking with the patient, and letting somebody else look at the blood and urine or count the cells in the spinal fluid—especially if that person (or machine) can work more rapidly and accurately than the physician himself.

One can argue that this presages a split among physicians, between those with a scientific, research orientation, and those with a behavioral, almost psychiatric, orientation. That split has already begun and some bemoan it. But, in reality, art and science have rarely merged well in a single individual. It is said that Einstein would have starved as a cellist, and it is certainly true that the number of doctors in recent years who have been both superb clinicians and excellent laboratory researchers is really quite small. Such men certainly can be found, and they are always impressive— but they are distinctly in the minority. In fact, the modern notion that the average physician is a practitioner of both art and science is at best a charming myth, at worst a serious occupational delusion.

✠

In the final analysis, what does all this mean for the hospital and for the patient in the hospital? One may look at the short-term possibilities, as represented by the burns treatment program.

It will reduce the mundane work of ward personnel, both doctors and nurses, and leave them more time to spend with the patient. For doctors, it should mean more time for research as well. And for the patient, that should ultimately be a good thing.

Furthermore, as an extension of the hospital, a computer program offers quite extraordinary possibilities. Any hospital in the country—or even any doctor's office —could utilize the program, by using existing telephone lines. A community hospital could plug into the MGH program and let the computer monitor the patient and direct therapy. As a way to utilize the innovative capability of the hospital, and its vast resources of complex medical information, this must surely represent a logical step in 2,500 years of evolution. And for the patient, that, too, should ultimately be a good thing.

EDITH MURPHY

Six months before she came to the MGH, Mrs. Murphy, a fifty-five-year-old mother of three, began to notice swelling of her legs and ankles. This swelling increased and she became progressively weaker, until finally she had to quit her job as a filing clerk. She consulted her local doctor, who prescribed digitalis and diuretics. This reduced the swelling but did not eliminate it completely. She continued to feel very weak.

Finally she was admitted to a local community hospital where she was found to be severely anemic, to have bleeding in her gastrointestinal tract, to have chemical evidence of liver disease, and X rays suggestive of cancer of the pancreas. At this point, she was transferred to the MGH. She knew nothing of her suspected diagnosis.

On arrival she was seen by Edmund Carey, a medical student, and Dr. A. W. Nienhuis, a house officer. They found that she was slightly jaundiced and that her abdomen was distended with fluid. Her liver could not be felt because of this fluid. Her legs and ankles were still swollen. They confirmed the presence of blood in her stools.

Laboratory studies indicated a hematocrit of 18 per cent, which meant that she had less than half the normal number of red blood cells. Her reticulocyte count, a measure of new-blood-cell production, was increased. A measurement of iron in her blood showed that she was iron-deficient. The total picture was thus consistent with chronic anemia from blood loss through the gastrointestinal tract,* but the situation was more complex: A Coombs blood test was positive, suggesting that her body was also destroying red cells by an allergic mechanism.

A chest X ray and electrocardiogram and kidney studies were normal. Barium X-ray studies of the upper GI tract, to check the suggestion of pancreatic cancer, could not be done immediately. A bone-marrow biopsy was done, but it gave no further clue to the nature of the anemia. Her abdomen was tapped and a sample of fluid withdrawn for analysis. There was laboratory evidence to suggest liver disease and perhaps insufficient

* The technical reader must excuse some simplification in this presentation.

proteins in her blood, but this could not be immediately confirmed on the night of admission.

Mrs. Murphy thus presented a complex and puzzling problem. The first question was whether a single disease process could explain her three major difficulties, which Dr. Nienhuis summarized as anemia, gastrointestinal disease, and edema. As he noted, they could all be explained, in whole or in part, by cancer or liver disease, by invoking mechanisms that are quite complicated.

Implicit in his thinking was the notion that the body is constantly changing, and that those features of the body which appear static are really the product of a dynamic equilibrium. Thus the red-cell volume of the body, which usually appears fairly constant, is really the product of ceaseless creation and destruction of cells. The average red cell has a life span of 120 days; anemia can result from either inadequate production of cells or excessive destruction of cells. In Mrs. Murphy's case, production seemed actually increased, but she was losing cells through bleeding and allergic destruction.

Similarly, water, which normally accounts for 70 per cent of body weight, is carefully distributed in a healthy person—so much inside cells, so much outside cells. Individual water molecules are constantly shifting around the body, but the balance in each compartment is closely maintained. Edema, the pathological swelling of certain tissues with water, can be caused by a wide range of factors that disrupt the normal distribution of body water. The same effect can be produced by heart disease, liver disease, or kidney disease, each by a different mechanism.

Mrs. Murphy was admitted to the Bulfinch medical wards and passed an uneventful night. In the morning she was seen on work rounds by Carey, Nienhuis, and another resident, Dr. Robert Liss. Practical aspects of her condition were discussed, particularly the question of transfusion. It was decided to postpone transfusion since she appeared comfortable for the moment. Later in the day Mrs. Murphy's problems were discussed with the visiting senior physician on the wards, Dr. John Mills. He felt that "tumor in the abdomen was strongly indicated," but for a variety of reasons felt that lymphoma, a cancer of lymph glands, was more likely than pancreatic cancer.

That same day, a radioactive liver scan was done to determine the size of the liver, since it could not be felt directly. The liver was found to be small and shrunken, suggestive of scarring from cirrhosis. The basis for this cirrhosis was unclear. Mrs. Murphy maintained that she was a non-drinker. She had no history of hepatitis in the past, and no occupational exposure to liver poisons. The cirrhosis was therefore labeled "cryptogenic," meaning of hidden cause.

For the next three days the question of cancer, or liver disease, or both, was widely discussed. As evidence of liver damage accumulated, cryptogenic* cirrhosis became the favored diagnostic possibility.

---

* To an outsider, the tendency among physicians to call certain diseases cryptogenic or idiopathic—and then to discuss them as if they

Meanwhile, Mrs. Murphy began to feel better. She received a transfusion of three units of blood, and felt better still. She did not, however, receive any further therapy.

Everyone agreed that a liver biopsy would be useful, but the patient had a bleeding tendency—presumably secondary to liver disease—which made a biopsy impossible. Other diagnostic procedures were not helpful. Sigmoidoscopy and barium enema failed to determine the origin of gastrointestinal bleeding. A check for cancer cells in her abdominal fluid was negative.

On the seventh hospital day, she was seen by Dr. Alexander Leaf, who suggested thyroid tests as well as tests for collagen diseases. The following day, Dr. Nienhuis raised the question of whether this patient might have lupoid hepatitis, a rare and somewhat disputed clinical entity.

In the next forty-eight hours, two important pieces of evidence were obtained. First, an upper GI series was done, and it was normal. There was no sign of cancer of the pancreas.

Second, a re-examination of the patient's white cells revealed several with large, abnormal, bluish lumps imbedded within the cell substance. These cells are called

---

were well-defined, understood clinical entities—may be perplexing. But in fact it serves a purpose. For one thing, it excludes diagnoses: anyone who speaks of cryptogenic cirrhosis has excluded alcoholic or posthepatitic cirrhosis. By implication, the term conveys more information than a simple "We don't know why." In the same way, idiopathic hypertension implies prior exclusion of the few known causes of this condition.

LE cells, for they are virtually diagnostic of a collagen disease, systemic lupus erythematosus.

This is a disease of enormous interest to physicians at the present time. Once considered rare, it is now seen with increasing frequency as diagnostic tests become more refined. Classically it has been considered a disease of middle-aged women, characterized by protean manifestations—fever, skin eruptions, and involvement of many other organs, particularly joints and kidneys. However, as lupus is better understood, the classical description is changing: more males are now found with SLE, and the range of clinical manifestations has broadened.

Lupus is called a collagen disease because it shares with certain other diseases a tendency to alter blood vessels and connective tissue, and because it seems, like these other diseases, to be caused by some form of hypersensitivity (allergy). This question of causation is by no means clear, but patients with the disease certainly show a wide variety of biochemical disorders of the immune system; lupus is frequently called "the auto-immune disease par excellence."

Normally, the body's immune mechanism produces antibodies to fight foreign agents, such as invading bacteria. This response is generally beneficial to the individual, although much recent work has gone into suppressing the response so that foreign organs can be transplanted.

However, it is now recognized that the body's natural

rejection mechanism can sometimes be mistakenly directed toward the body itself. In some way the individual's capacity to distinguish what is native from what is foreign is disrupted; the patient attempts to produce immunity to himself—and proceeds to attack certain of his own tissues, leading to "a chronic civil war within the body."

In the case of lupus, the patient produces several sorts of antibodies against himself. One of these attacks DNA, the genetic substance of chromosomes. This damaged DNA is later ingested by white cells, producing the characteristic bluish lumps. However, SLE patients also produce other auto-antibodies, which are seen in other conditions. Thus Mrs. Murphy was found to have anti-DNA antibodies, increased gamma globulin, and antibodies against thyroid, as well as antibodies found in rheumatoid arthritis.

Immune disorders as a cause or complication of illness are now suspected for a great range of diseases, including rheumatic fever, pernicious anemia, myasthenia gravis, multiple sclerosis, Hashimoto's thyroiditis, and glomerulonephritis. Immune and auto-immune mechanisms are thus of considerable interest; investigation of these mechanisms represents one of the major thrusts of current medical research.

For systemic lupus erythematosus, however, there is no cure and no good information on prognosis. Patients have died within a few months of onset; others have lived fifteen or twenty years. For Mrs. Murphy, therapy consisted of diuretics, which resulted in loss of thirty-two pounds of fluid, and a cautious trial of corticosteroids to suppress some effects of the disease. She was discharged feeling well and returned to her job.

✠

The case of Mrs. Murphy illustrates an important function of the ward patient in the university hospital that differentiates him from the private patient: the ward patient is there in part to help turn students into doctors. For the patient, this has its drawbacks as well as its advantages.

First, to clarify some terms:

A medical student is anyone with a bachelor's degree who is in the midst of four years of graduate work leading to the M.D. degree, but not yet to a license to practice. To be licensed, he must spend an additional year as an intern in a teaching hospital.

An intern is thus anyone with an M.D. who is in his first year out of medical school. An intern is licensed to practice only within the hospital. After a year of internship, he could theoretically leave and begin private practice, but practically nobody does. Instead, interns go on to become residents.

A resident is anyone who has finished his internship and is continuing with more specialized training in such areas as pediatrics, surgery, internal medicine, or psychiatry. A residency may be taken at the same hospital as the internship or at another; residencies last from two to six years, depending on the field.

Medical students are primarily responsible to the medical school, not the hospital; within the hospital they are referred to, somewhat ironically, as "studs."

Interns and residents, on the other hand, are hospital employees and are referred to as "house officers." Collectively, the interns and residents comprise the "house staff," as distinct from the "senior staff," meaning the private physicians or academic teachers affiliated with the hospital.

This hierarchy is analogous to a university with its undergraduates, graduate students, and professors. There are departments within the hospital corresponding to university departments; these departments give courses for medical students and house officers, termed "rotations." Primarily, the teaching is informal, but there is also a heavy schedule of formal rounds, lectures, and seminars.

In the history of the teaching hospital, as in the university, the undergraduate (or medical student) appeared much earlier than the graduate student (or house officer). Indeed, the beginnings of the teaching hospitals are closely associated with the beginnings of medical schools in this country. This was clearly the case for the first three medical schools, and the first three teaching hospitals in America: in Philadelphia, New York, and Boston.

The Massachusetts General had Harvard students on

the wards from its inception. There is no reason to believe the students made the hospital more appealing; Warren recalled that students in his day "were of the crudest character," and remembers that it was no recommendation to a landlady to say you were a medical student. Even a century later, Harvey Cushing grumbled that "students in a hospital, like children in a lodging house, are not an unmixed blessing." But despite persistent reservations, the teaching hospital has always taught medical students. What is new is the teaching of house officers.

Originally, medical students were required to take two years of academic courses, followed by a third year as an apprentice to a practicing physician. In those days the MGH had two house officer positions—then known by the considerably more humble term "house pupils" —and these posts were acceptable substitutes for an apprenticeship. Beginning around the time of the Civil War, however, the hospital began to expand its house-officer posts; the greatest growth came at the turn of the century. In 1891, there were seven house officers; by 1901, fourteen; by 1911, twenty-one. As mentioned, there are now 304.

Part of this growth represents a simple growth of the hospital. As it became larger, there were more patients to care for, and to learn from, and more day-to-day work to be done by house officers.

Part of the growth represents the increasing role of the hospital as an acute-care facility. The hospital sees fewer patients with chronic diseases and more acutely ill patients who require continuous and careful management. This requires a larger house staff.

Partly, too, the growth represents a shift away from the old personal apprentice system toward an "institutional apprenticeship." In the 1930's and 1940's, it became clear that house officers who remained in the hospital were better trained than those who left early and linked up with private practitioners. This observation finally led to virtual abandonment of the personal apprenticeship. Thus, formerly, surgical residency was three years, followed by two years of apprenticeship under a private man; now it is five years (including internship), and the only reason for joining a private surgeon at the end of that time is to build a practice, not to gain more experience.

All this means that the structure of patient care is quite different today from what it was when the hospital first opened. In 1821, patient care was essentially in the hands of private, senior men who donated their time to the hospital and agreed to take students around with them on the wards. But between student and senior man there has sprung up a large body of individuals who are now essential to the functioning of the hospital. The MGH could cheerfully dispense with its medical students, but it would come to a grinding halt in a few hours if deprived of its house staff.

It is no exaggeration to say that the house staff runs large areas of the hospital, with senior men advising from above, and students looking on from below. One may applaud this system for providing a spectrum of competence and responsibility, allowing students to move up the ladder to internship, then junior and senior residency, in easy stages. But in fact the emergence and proliferation of house officers has another, much harsher rationale. For the hospital, they provide a source of trained, intelligent, hard-working, very cheap labor.

This has always been true. In 1896, when Cushing was an intern, he noted that "house officers are about as hard worked men as I have ever seen. Every day is twenty-four hours long for them with a vengeance."

The modern house officer generally works an "every other night" schedule, meaning roughly thirty-six hours on duty, and twelve off. In practice this means arriving at the hospital at six thirty or seven in the morning, working all day and probably most of the night, continuing through the following day until late afternoon, and then going home to sleep—until six thirty or seven the next day. Payment for this effort, which is sustained over many years, was until quite recently nonexistent. Some hospitals were so bad that they worked their house officers at this pace, paid them nothing, and charged them for laundry and parking. Others would provide a few meals, and perhaps an honorarium fee of twenty-five dollars a year. At the MGH, a senior man recalls that as recently as ten years ago, "I was chief resident in surgery, eight years out of medical school, having spent two year in the army; I had a wife and four children; I was responsible for the conduct of an entire surgical service—and I was paid just under two thousand dollars a year."

Such a situation requires either an independent income or a great tolerance for debt; one wonders whether the modern stereotype of the private physician as crassly avaricious can be traced back to these years of early, absurd financial hardship. Fortunately, the salaries of house officers have climbed sharply in recent years. In many hospitals an intern now receives six thousand dollars, a senior resident eight or nine. Many factors are responsible for the increase: the effect of Medicare, which permits the hospital to charge patients for the services of a resident; the fact that the G.I. bill has been extended to cover residency training; the realization among medical educators that you cannot get and keep good people in an affluent society without paying them.

As the house officers have become more numerous and more skilled, the position of the medical student has changed. House officers are licensed to practice medicine; students cannot practice by law. A student cannot write orders, even for something as simple as raising a patient's bed, without having them countersigned by a house officer.

Legally, a student is permitted to employ nothing other than diagnostic instruments, and then only for the purpose of diagnosis. In practice, this ruling is stretched to mean that a student can, under supervision, perform a lumbar puncture, a thoracic or abdominal tap, or a bone-marrow aspirate; he can suture wounds in the emergency ward; he can also mix medicines, start intravenous infusions, inject medicines intravenously, and give a blood transfusion. Additionally, he is expected to have competence in a variety of laboratory procedures and tests.

The medical student's officially sanctioned functions thus lie somewhere between those of a doctor, a nurse, and a laboratory technician. It is not surprising that no one knows what to call him. Instructors with a group of second- or third-year students will often introduce them to patients as "doctors in training" or "these young doctors." Fourth-year students, seeing patients alone, will introduce themselves as "doctor." Until a few years ago, the students even wore name tags which said "Dr. ———," but this practice was abandoned after the hospital was advised it constituted misrepresentation that might have legal consequences. Student name tags now give only their names; those of interns and residents say "Dr."

It is not clear why medical students are called doctors in front of patients, especially since so few patients are fooled by the appellation. One can view the whole business as a harmless convention, in which the hospital pretends that its students are doctors, and the patients pretend to be taken in.

Why bother? Instructors say that this small white lie comforts the patients, who would be upset to learn they were being examined by students. Something of the same sort happens with interns, who occasionally pass themselves off as residents in the belief that this soothes patients. It is true that the folklore—and the mass-media image—of the medical student and the intern is distinctly unfavorable, and these negative connotations persist until residency. (Dr. Kildare, that charming, all-knowing physician, was a resident who spent much prime time dealing with neurotic, guilt-ridden, fumbling interns and students.) "Even now," according to George Orwell, "doctors can be found whose motives are questionable. Anyone who has had much illness, or who has listened to medical students talking, will know what I mean." In a single, paradoxical stroke, he dismisses the motivations of *some* doctors, but *all* medical students.

The position of the medical student is thus peculiar, and occasionally comical. In society at large, he finds himself eminently marriageable and a good credit risk, thus enjoying the approval of those two bastions of conservative appraisal—matrons and bankers. In the hospital, however, those same matrons and bankers want nothing to do with students, and nearly every student has had the experience of examining a woman who grumbles and complains throughout the history and physical and then politely asks if the student is married.

In the end, one suspects that the practice of labeling students as doctors is misguided. Patients ought to be told explicitly who the students are; a moment's reflection shows many advantages to such a practice.

For one thing, most patients coming into a teaching

hospital are already apprehensive about being used as guinea pigs. They have heard vague reports that "You'll be in the hands of students and interns," and this is not really true. Patients entering the hospital—already sick and afraid—are almost always unfamiliar with the hierarchy of decision-making that provides careful checks on junior men. Against this background of apprehension is added the fact that everyone introduces himself as a doctor, while the patient knows perfectly well that some of those doctors are students. Thus, failure to identify students increases anxiety instead of relieving it.

Further, it is a common observation on the wards that students are popular with patients. Students have more time to talk to patients; hospital life for a patient is boring; patients like the attention. (Frequently they will rank the house staff according to warmth and attentiveness. A friendly student who has had the experience of working with a brusque resident knows how often patients conclude that the resident is a student, and vice versa.*)

Finally, it is explicit in the bargain any teaching hospital makes that a patient will receive better care, but in return must put up with teaching. The teaching function might as well be identified as such. In any case, as Frederick Cheever Shattuck said many years ago, "Before swerving from or denying the truth we should ask ourselves the searching question, 'For whose advantage

---

* This implies that patients associate brusqueness with professional ineptitude, and that may be valid.

is this denial?' If it is in any measure for our advantage, or seeming advantage, let us shame the devil."

✠

How do students, house officers, and senior men combine to produce the ward teaching system? As exemplified by Mrs. Murphy's experience, the system works as follows.

When the ward is notified that a new patient is being admitted, the student goes down to the EW and examines the patient. On occasion, he has to hurry to beat the house officer, but students learn to do this, and the best house officers will go to great lengths to allow the student to perform the initial examination. The reason for this is that with each succeeding history and physical, the patient becomes more accustomed to the routine of delivering his story in an orderly but unnatural manner. Fresh patients are the most difficult to get a history from, and therefore the most prized.

After a student has examined the patient, the resident conducts a second examination, and then comes out to talk to the student about the case. The resident generally has only three questions: "What did you find?" "What do you think he has?" "What do you want to do for him?" Interestingly, these are the only really important questions in all clinical medicine.

A discussion of diagnosis and treatment follows; if the resident agrees with the student, he will let him

write the orders, then countersign them. Diagnostic procedures such as lumbar puncture, bone-marrow biopsy,
and so on are usually done by the student under the
resident's supervision. By tradition, patients are expected to be "worked up" as much as possible on the day
(or night) of admission. This means that in addition to
the history and physical, the ward team is supposed to
look at the blood morphology, do a white cell count, a
hematocrit, an electrocardiogram, urinalysis, review the
chest X ray—and whatever other, more sophisticated,
tests are necessary, all on the night of admission.

The student may do much or all of this, but he really
has no control over the patient's care. Most of the decisions—decisions at the time of admission, and all later
decisions—are made by the admitting house officer. This
is why the medical service regards "admitting a patient" as directly equivalent to the surgeon's "doing a
case." In each instance, only one person can have the
responsibility of decisions on patient care. And while
it is valuable to look on, it is not the same thing as
doing it yourself. The experience of responsibility is
not transferable.

Each house officer thus has a series of "his patients"
on the ward; these are the patients he originally admitted, and he feels primary responsibility for them
throughout their hospital stay. He is expected to know
more about his patients than anyone else, though others
must know enough to handle details of care when the
resident is off duty. The sense of individual responsibil-

ity is so strong that it is couched in possessive terms. One house officer may ask another, "Is Mr. Jones your patient?" and be told, "No, he's Bob's."

The student's role in all this is to pretend that he is the admitting house officer, and to continue pretending so throughout the hospital stay. A student generally works closely with one intern or resident, keeping the same hours, following him along. Among students there is an active grapevine to keep everyone informed about which house officers are good to work with and which not. A good house officer is one who is confident of his skill (insecurity is catching); willing to take time to teach the student; and unwilling to delegate all routine work, termed "scut," to the student.

On the morning after a patient's admission, during "work rounds" from 7:45 to 9:00, when the ward team goes from patient to patient, the student is expected to summarize informally the history, physical, and lab tests for the benefit of those team members who were off duty the previous night. A formal discussion is given by the student during "visit rounds" later in the day, when he relates the details of the case to the visiting physician, usually just called "the visit." The visit is a staff members of the hospital, assigned to the wards for a month, and legally responsible for all the patients on the ward.

The student's formal discussion is known as "presenting." To present a patient means to deliver the salient information in a brief, highly stylized form. The student is expected to do this from memory. A presentation begins with events leading up to admission for the present illness; then goes on to past medical history; then a review of organ systems; family and social history; physical findings beginning at the head and working down to the feet. Laboratory data is then presented in a specific order: blood studies, urine studies, cardiogram, X rays, and finally more specialized tests.

The entire process is not supposed to take more than five minutes.

A good presentation is difficult, for along with summarizing positive findings, the student is expected to include certain "pertinent negatives" from among the almost infinite number of symptoms and signs the patient does *not* have. These pertinent negatives are intended to exclude specific diagnoses. Thus, if a patient has jaundice and a large liver, the student should state that the patient does not drink, if this is the case.

Aggressive students can be quite abstruse in their negatives, hoping that the instructor will interrupt and ask (for example): "What were you thinking when you said the patient had never danced in Tibet?"

To this the student can triumphantly name some obscure disease that vaguely fits the situation, such as "the Kurelu Dancing Syndrome, sir." He thus appears well read. The game can be dangerous with a knowledgeable visit, however, for he is likely to shoot back: "The Kurelu Dancing Syndrome never occurs in males under forty, and your patient is thirty-six. If you want to do some reading, I refer you to the *Kurelu Medical Journal*, volume ten, number two." This is a signal for the student to crumble; he has lost the round—unless, of course, he has a rejoinder. There is only one acceptable form: "But, sir, in the *Mauritanian Journal of Midwifery* last week there was a report of a case in a ten-year-old boy." This may, or may not, work. The visit may reply, "The *what* journal? Wasn't that the one which reported that skimmed milk caused cancer?"

That ends the discussion.

Among students, visits are classified into two groups— "benign," and the others. It depends on how the visits treat students. Generally the visit sits in silence throughout the presentation; he then begins by pointing out all the things the student forgot to mention; and then proceeds to ask questions. He is entitled to ask questions on anything he likes, so long as it vaguely relates to the case at hand. He can, if he wishes, keep the student hopping.

For example, a typical discussion about a case of stress duodenal ulcer might have the visit first asking the anatomy of the four parts of the duodenum; then the arterial supply to the stomach; the common complications of duodenal ulcer; the factors that classically increase and decrease ulcer pain; the features that distinguish ulcer pain from the pain of acute pancreatitis, gall bladder disease, or heart attack; the four indications for surgical intervention; the reasons for measuring serum pancreatic amylase and serum calcium; the mental changes one might expect with GI bleeding in the presence of liver disease, and the reason for the change; the other causes of upper GI bleeding; the way to distinguish upper and lower GI bleeding, and so on.

Furthermore, the visit can shift to a related topic at any point. If he asks about serum calcium and the student correctly answers that there is a relation between parathyroid disease and ulcer, the visit may go on to ask how calcium fluctuates in parathyroid disease; the associated changes in serum phosphate; what changes might be seen in the electrocardiogram; what mental changes are associated with increased and decreased serum calcium, in adults and in children.

Thus a student who began talking about ulcer disease is effectively shunted to calcium metabolism. And, at any time, the visit can turn around, demand to know six other conditions associated with ulcer,* and go on to discuss each of them. Visit rounds are two hours long. There is plenty of time.

For the most part, interns and residents are exempt from grilling; it is considered too undignified. The visit treats house officers as colleagues, but not students. A house officer who asks a question of the visit will get an answer. A student who asks a question will most often get a question back, as in "Sir, what does the serum calcium do in Chicken Little disease?" "Well, what do the

---

* Such as chronic lung disease, cirrhosis, rheumatoid arthritis, burns and strokes, pancreatitis, and the effects of cetain drug therapies, especially steroids.

plasma proteins do in Ridinghood's Macroglobulin-
emia?" If the student fails to see the light, he will get
another hint, also in the form of a question: "Well, then,
what about the serum phosphate in Heavyweight's
Syndrome?"

This is a form of a game which is repeated over and
over again in medical teaching. It is a game useful to the
conduct of medical practice. A very simple example of
the game is the following:

STUDENT: "The patient has a rash and fever."
VISIT: "Has he ever been to Martha's Vineyard?"
STUDENT: "No, he does not have Rocky Mountain
spotted fever."

The point is that the student sees the implication behind the question—that each year one or two cases of
Rocky Mountain spotted fever are contracted on Martha's Vineyard. Such deductive processes are precisely
those important to the conduct of medicine, and therefore represent a useful teaching method. In the extreme,
this can lead to a leap-frog interchange which is almost
beyond the understanding of the casual observer:

STUDENT: "The patient has kidney disease consistent
with glomerulonephritis."
VISIT: "Was there a recent history of infection?"
STUDENT: "Anti-streptolysin titers were low."
VISIT: "Was there a facial rash?"

STUDENT: "LE prep and anti-nuclear antibodies were negative."

VISIT: "Were there eyeground changes?"

STUDENT: "Glucose-tolerance test was normal."

VISIT: "Did you consider rectal biopsy?"

STUDENT: "The tongue was not enlarged."

This is jumping from mountaintop to mountaintop, skipping the valleys. In translation, the visit is asking, first, whether the glomerulonephritis was caused by streptococcal infection; second, whether it is due to lupus; third, to diabetes; and finally, whether due to amyloidosis. The student is denying each diagnosis by presenting negative data. Neither teacher nor student specifies the diagnosis; the game is to figure out what each is talking about without saying what it is.

This Socratic tradition of teaching medical students dates back to the days when medicine was an apprenticeship in the strictest sense. The Socratic method has the virtue of informality: on work rounds, the resident can ask the student in passing, "How will we know when Mr. Jones is adequately digitalized?" and the surgeon can pause in his operation to ask the student, "What would happen if I cut this nerve here?" It is a good way to keep the student constantly recirculating his knowledge through his brain, and by and large it works well.

Why not just state the fact, as a declarative statement, for the edification of the student? There is just one major reason: most medical students are tired. At any given moment, a lecture to a medical student is a signal to click off, to tune out, to go to sleep. Partly, this is a learned response. It is common, during the first two years of medical school, to have four hours of lectures and five hours of laboratory work in a single day. Students who are studying late into the night on top of this schedule learn to sleep during lectures with great facility. The pattern carries on into the clinical years. One can observe lectures to medical students and house staff in the hospital in which 20 to 50 per cent of the class is slumped over in their chairs. The lecturer pays no attention. To a lecturer, it is not an insult, but a fact of life. Everybody accepts it; everybody expects it.

The only way to beat the dozing off is to ask questions. Supposedly this makes the learning experience more active, less passive. But, as anyone who has ever attempted to put together a programmed text knows, teaching by questions is extraordinarily difficult. The ideal set of questions is graded, going from fact to fact, leading the student from information he knows well to the reasoning out of information he does not know. On the other hand, the usual unplanned set of questions just draws a blank look and a guess.

For some reason, the question-and-answer teaching method is a peculiarity of professional school instruction. It is common in law, medicine, and business, and practically unknown in other graduate fields. The best teachers can employ it to great effect; most teachers are hopeless at it.

The system is most likely to succeed when applied to an individual—and almost certain to fail when applied to large groups. I have watched a specialist in diabetes walk into a room full of third-year students, rub his hands together, and say: "All right. Let's suppose you've gotten your diabetic patient. He has a blood sugar of three hundred. What kind of diet are you going to put him on?" Nobody in the room had the faintest idea what kind of diet to put him on. "How many grams of carbohydrate do you want to give him?" the instructor demanded. Nobody knew; nobody said anything. Finally he pointed to a student and insisted on a figure. "Ninety grams?" the student said. "Wrong!" said the instructor, and went around the room until somebody finally guessed one hundred grams, the figure he wanted to hear. "Now then, how much insulin do you want to start him with?" the instructor asked, and the game began again.

It would be pleasant to think such examples atypical of medical education, but in fact they are more the rule than the exception. Considerable dedication is required of students to learn medicine in the face of such teaching; one often has the impression that medical education works despite itself.

Useful changes can be made in all elements of the process—changes in the students, changes in the teachers, changes in the teaching methodology. Of these, only one appears very likely: the traditional routine of every-other-night for clinical students and house officers is dying. Many hospitals are shifting to an every-third-night schedule, which makes a considerable difference. The student or house officer sleeps through his first night off, but he is able to read during the second night; and during the day he is more alert, more awake. This helps to remove one of the oldest paradoxes in medical education—namely that the hospital claims to provide an excellent learning environment, while systematically depriving its students of sleep.

A change in teachers is less likely. Clinical teaching posts have status attached to them; a private man likes to be able to say he "spends some time with the students." At the same time, teaching hasn't got much value as a way to be promoted within the academic hierarchy; medicine, like every other field, puts its emphasis on published research. This leads to a multitude of rather casual teachers who may spend only a few hours a year with the students. These people—like the diabetes expert, who comes to the hospital once every three months to deliver his little talk—are most pernicious. They do not care enough about teaching to attempt to do it well; they don't have enough experience with students to know how to direct their talk; they have never received any training in exposition and attach no significance to a good delivery.

Having dismissed these people, one should say that medicine does indeed correctly sense that private, experienced practitioners have accumulated practical knowledge that ought to be communicated to students. Unfortunately, this is not the way to do it.

Methods of teaching require considerable revision. You can be assured that this is taking place—it is always taking place and always has been. Curricula change, new courses spring up and others die, grand lectures on education are given citing Cushing and Osler, but somehow the fundamental quality of medical education remains the same.

The methodology continues to be perplexing. The notion that the subject should be suited to the manner of teaching; the idea that certain things are best taught in lectures, others in seminars, others individually; the understanding of those qualities that distinguish the lecture from the slide from the printed page from the visceral experience—all these things are traditionally lacking in medicine.

Future medical educators, for example, will probably look back on the teaching hospital and shake their heads at the way "patient material" was used. One can argue that this use, at the present time, is highly inefficient. The individual patient in a teaching hospital is not intensively used for teaching. A bizarre case may be seen by fifty or sixty people, but the average ward patient is seen by many fewer, particularly if his problem is common and his stay in the hospital is short.

The need to see patients firsthand is an important part of medical education; one must have experience with many ill individuals, exhibiting many different manifestations of disease. This is necessary because there are both many diseases, and many forms that a disease will take in different people. To obtain the proper depth and breadth of experience requires a long time; a student or house officer must remain in the hospital at all hours for many years. Otherwise, he is going to miss vital experiences.

However, a number of ways of "saving the patient for future reference" are now possible. Teaching collections of X rays have existed for several years, enabling students to gain broad radiological experience without waiting for the patients actually to come in. But this is only the beginning: one can record a patient's appearance and important physical findings on video tape; one can even record an interview and history-taking. By such techniques literally hundreds of students can, over a period of years, have some experience with a given patient.

And one can go further. For example, one of the most severe limitations of modern clinical teaching is that the student cannot really use the patient to "practice on." While mistakes are an important part in any learning process, in the hospital they are discouraged and guarded against—and rightly so.

What is needed, of course, is a disposable patient, for whom mistakes do not matter. In the past, one can argue, the disposable patient was provided by society in the form of the charity case (at least this was the popular belief); but this requirement can now be provided by technology. Anesthetists have developed a lifelike plastic dummy patient for students to practice on; this dummy can have allergic reactions to anesthesia, cardiac and respiratory arrests, and a variety of other serious complications. The student can practice on the dummy with impunity. So far, the only analogous situation is that provided by the post-mortem patient who is used for practice of surgical procedure. But we will see much more in the future.

For example, a teaching program can be put on a computer, enabling the student to ask the "patient" questions, and get back replies. On the basis of such an interview, the student can make a diagnosis and institute therapy. The computer can then inform the student of the consequences of his prescribed regimen.

In fact, such methods are already in use in the National Board Examinations, Part III—the section given to interns prior to certification. The exam contains, among other things, film clips of patients, followed by questions about the patient's disease. It also contains a most interesting section consisting of brief histories, followed by specific questions, such as "What would you do immediately for this patient?" After each question is a series of possible answers, such as "Begin intravenous fluid replacement," "Start antibiotics," "Give digitalis," and so on. And following each answer is a blacked-out space.

The student selects the therapy he wants and erases the blacked-out space to reveal the consequences of his choice. If he has chosen correctly, the answer will be encouraging: "Patient improves." But if he is wrong, the answer is likely to be a harsh "Patient dies."

Using these techniques, it is possible to give the student exposure to rare clinical situations he might never see otherwise. It is also possible to give the student exposure in depth to a problem. One could program the differing clinical histories of a dozen patients with hyperthyroidism, for example, and let the student work through them all, to get some idea of the differences from case to case.

None of this will ever replace experience at the bedside, but it will certainly supplement that experience— and very soon. There are two reasons why such techniques will gain rapid acceptance.

The first is a slowly simmering rebellion against the length of medical education. In this country the average physician is almost halfway to the grave before he is prepared to start practice—and the trend is toward even longer educational periods, not shorter ones. At the same time, there is a demand for more physicians, and the suggestion that this demand can be met, in part, by faster education. There is also a growing suspicion that in affluent America some of the best young men shun medicine because the educational period is so long.

As an educational process, medicine has suffered the full effects of the scientific outpouring of information; the response of medical educators has been simplistic— to lengthen the period of formal training as the body of knowledge has increased. This cannot go on indefinitely, and specialization—breaking up knowledge into smaller and smaller areas—will not provide the whole solution.

As a stopgap measure, medical schools have kept the total number of years constant, but have lengthened the per-week teaching load. Thus medical students at Harvard attend twice as many hours of classes per week as law or business students. Of necessity, this makes medical education a very passive business and deprives the student of the single most important thing he desperately needs to learn while at school—how to initiate the educational process for himself, later on, when he is a practitioner.

For medical schools there are only two solutions: to teach less or to teach more efficiently. Medicine has been reluctant—sometimes wisely, sometimes not—to teach less. Curriculum changes are a traditional sport, but they occur slowly (John Foster notes that "it is easier to move a graveyard than to change a medical curriculum") and never seem to make manageable the total information to be mastered. The current administrative structure of medical schools appears incapable of curtailing the curriculum. Educators must therefore devise ways to teach faster. It is the only solution.

If it is hard to be a student, it is much harder to be a good visit, for a visiting physician has the most difficult teaching job in the world. His "class" of students, interns, and residents is small, but their depth of knowledge is dissimilar, and the visit must endeavor to teach everyone. His subject matter is all of medical knowledge; he must act simultaneously as adviser, librarian, lecturer, and, at the bedside, as a direct example in dealing with patients. The best visit is a marvel to watch. In an hour he can listen to the student, quiz him, arrive at a diagnosis, proceed to deliver a ten-minute extemporaneous lecture on some aspect of the diagnosis, throw in one or two humorous anecdotes, see the patient and elicit more information than the students and house staff were able to obtain, in the process demonstrate an obscure physical sign, then step into the hall and summarize the entire situation in a few minutes.

And then go on to the second patient of the day.

The whole act depends on vast knowledge, clear organization, boundless energy. But it is also the final check in the long system of built-in checks—the intern checks on the student, the resident checks on the intern, and the visit checks on everybody.

What does all this mean for the patient? Most teaching hospital physicians believe it produces better patient care. According to Dr. Robert Ebert, dean of Harvard Medical School, "It is far easier to check on the mistakes of an incompetent intern than the mistakes of an incompetent private physician. It is one of the ironies of our system of medicine that a very sick charity patient in the ward is likely to receive better and more constant medical attention than his counterpart on the private side of the hospital."

These considerations lead Dr. Ebert to talk of "the privileges of being used for teaching." This is an idea foreign to most private patients, yet our definition of the "teaching patient" is in the midst of drastic revision for that most fundamental of reasons, money. The financial structure of the hospital is changing, and with it, everything else.

Originally, the Massachusetts General and hospitals like it were founded to care for the sick *poor*. Patients entering the hospital agreed to be used for teaching, in exchange for medical care they could obtain no other way. At this time, there were virtually no private patients in the hospital. Any individual of means preferred to be treated—and to be operated on, if necessary—in his own home. Even at the turn of the century, the hospital was no place for the wealthy. When the Peter Bent Brigham Hospital was built in Boston in 1913, its planners made no provision for private patients.

Soon thereafter things began to change. The development of anesthesia made operations more common, and the use of Listerian antisepsis did much to reduce cross-infection and epidemics of "hospitalism." The hospital emerged as a place for all severely ill patients, private or charity cases alike. In 1917, the MGH built a pavilion entirely for private patients, and in 1930, another. By 1935, 40 per cent of hospital beds were occupied by paying patients. By 1955, it was nearly 50 per cent. In 1967, some 60 per cent of patients admitted to the hospital went to private pavilions.

Nor do these figures tell the whole story, for even on the wards, patients with no financial resources for medical care hardly exist. At present, 85 per cent of all MGH patients have some form of "third party" health coverage—and most of those who do not are very wealthy patients, not poor ones.

Third-party payment, whether by insurance plan such as Blue Cross, state welfare, or Medicare, has revolutionized the position of the teaching hospital. Put bluntly, it is no longer possible to trade free care for teaching; nearly everyone can pay for his care, and can afford a private doctor, and a private or semi-private room.

The MGH is, at this writing, closing down its wards. Some other hospitals have already done so. Such structural changes are relatively simple, but a major dilemma remains. There are no charity patients left, and no private patient wants to be a "teaching patient," since this has disagreeable connotations.

What is the solution? There are, obviously, only two answers. Either teaching is halted or private patients are used for teaching purposes. The first solution is impractical, the second highly controversial. But it is clearly in the cards: someday, all patients in a teaching hospital will be used for teaching. Such a program has already been set up at another Boston teaching hospital, the Beth Israel. There, "ward" and private patients lie side by side, and all patients, whether they have private physicians or not, receive their in-hospital treatment from house staff.

Now all this may seem like a minor matter. After all, just 2 per cent of American hospitals are teaching hospitals. The rest have no such problem. But one may ask, if the teaching hospital truly delivers better medical care—if this claim is more than a rationalization for making private patients available for poking and prodding by medical students and interns—then shouldn't all hospitals adopt the methods of the teaching hospital? Shouldn't all patients have the benefits of the system?

There are some practical considerations, in terms of the availability of interns and residents, but we can ignore these and simply look more closely at the intrinsic quality, the advantages and disadvantages, of teaching patient care.

Certainly there are some classic advantages. The fact that residents are literally that—individuals residing in the hospital—means there are more doctors around, day and night, to treat acute emergencies. A patient with the finest private physician in the world will not be consoled if his doctor is away in his office when the patient has a cardiac arrest.

Second, as the pace of medical development accelerates, the hospital's staff of academicians and researchers can claim up-to-date, specialized information of a depth and variety that other hospitals, and individual private physicians, cannot hope to match. The impact of this on patient care can be considerable in some instances. For most of medical history, it did not matter whether your doctor was up to date or ten years behind the times; now it may matter if he is only one year behind. Therefore, one of the great new appeals of the teaching hospital is the availability of the most recent knowledge in patient care.

Third, the academic orientation of the staff leads them to attack perplexing problems with unusual vigor, reviewing the medical literature, utilizing the laboratory and referral resources of the institution. Endless rounds and discussions among house staff and visits mean that a problem will receive the benefit of many opinions. Thus a patient with an obscure disease or a difficult diagnosis will get a great deal of attention—much more than any single physician could give him.

Fourth, because the hospital is structured to teach and do research, it is critical of all medical practice, including its own. Each physician has several others looking over his shoulder, and this tends to minimize mistakes. To that extent a teaching patient is "safer" than a private patient.

All this is clearly evident when one looks at Mrs. Murphy's history. She is a patient with an uncommon, though not rare, disease—but a disease that manifested itself in an extraordinarily rare way. Mrs. Murphy first saw a private physician, who treated her complaint of swelling legs as if she had heart failure. She did not have heart failure. She did not improve. She then went to a community hospital, where more sophisticated tests were done. There, she was correctly found to have liver disease, GI bleeding, and hemolytic anemia. Each of these problems could have been discovered by her private doctor, with the help of a private clinical laboratory, but for reasons which cannot be assessed, he failed to do so.

At the community hospital, evidence was also found for pancreatic cancer. This evidence was incorrect. (Furthermore, important pathology unrelated to her primary disease was missed. This was not discussed in the earlier section, out of a desire to avoid complicating an already intricate story. However, in the report sent by the hospital to the MGH when the patient was admitted, a physical examination form clearly stated that a pelvic exam was normal. In fact, Mrs. Murphy had a cervical polyp the size of a large marble. It was easily felt and clearly visible. The only reasonable conclusion is that a pelvic examination was not, in fact, done at the other hospital.) And the only reason Mrs. Murphy was transferred to the MGH was because of this suspected diagnosis.

Two points about this story should be made immediately. The first is that the MGH, by its very nature, sees a great many patients whose diagnoses have been missed. It is easy to gain the impression that all practicing doctors are inept, and all community hospitals incompetent. But, in fact, the great majority of patients who receive correct diagnoses and good care never show up at the MGH.

Second, no medical system is perfect. Teaching hospitals make mistakes just the way community hospitals and private physicians do. Each teaching hospital in Boston delights in getting the patients of others, and making diagnoses that were missed. The point of Mrs. Murphy's story, therefore, is not the glorification of the teaching hospital, but rather that this woman, with a complex disease and unusual manifestations, received nine days of the most intense academic scrutiny before a diagnosis was established. She was immersed in an environment geared to such scrutiny. A great many people—from students to the chief of medicine—saw her, examined her, and contributed suggestions concerning her care. And from that eventually came a diagnosis that might not have been made otherwise.

At the same time, there are some classic complaints about teaching service care, from both patients and physicians. Patients dislike multiple examinations, and having to tell their story over and over again. Physicians complain that the academic orientation of a teaching service leads to excessive lab tests, too many diagnostic procedures, less briskly efficient care, longer in-hospital stays, and ultimately more expensive treatment. Without question, these complaints have some truth in them.

For example, it is relatively easy to dismiss the protests of a patient with an unknown disease who objects to many examinations by different people. It is in his own best interests to be examined by everyone, at least until a diagnosis is arrived at. However, it is less easy to shrug off the complaints of a patient who may have, unknown to him, a "classic case" of something that is neither rare nor unusual. An intelligent patient with a lucid history of ulcer may find himself visited by large number of students who are directed to him by an instructor who tells them, "Mr. Jones has a good story and good findings." And worse, if the patient complains to a resident, the resident cannot evaluate the complaint. No one keeps track of how many students are visiting any given patient. It is impossible to know whether he is objecting to two visits or to twenty.*

The question of excessive and unnecessary tests is difficult to evaluate. Everyone who works in a hospital sees patients who receive too many tests, under the guise of a "thorough work-up"; everyone has seen diagnostic procedures carried out where at least an element of motivation was the resident's desire to practice the procedure. These cases are rare, though they stick in one's mind.

Frequently, the issues can be subtle. They are polarized in the following verbatim exchange between a particularly obnoxious student and a particularly obnoxious visit. The patient under discussion was one who had

---

* Despite the above, most patients are not seen by many students. A fair percentage never set eyes on a student.

documented obstructive lung disease with advanced emphysema. He was on the respirator full time.

VISIT: "Do you think we should do cardiac catheterization and get a pulmonary wedge pressure on this man?"

STUDENT: "No."

VISIT: "Can you think of any additional information we might get from the wedge pressure?"

STUDENT: "No."

VISIT: "In point of fact, we know that in emphysema, if we find the wedge pressure elevated, then the severity of the disease is increased."

STUDENT: "Will that change your course of therapy?"

VISIT: "I'm not sure that's a valid consideration."

STUDENT: "There's a morbidity attached to pulmonary catheterization."

VISIT: "Yes, but it's very slight."

STUDENT: "It exists. If it won't change your therapy, how can you justify it?"

VISIT: "I don't think you can say it won't change our therapy."

STUDENT: "Then how might it change your therapy?"

VISIT: "Over the long haul. For instance, in this lab we do VD/VT measurements, though similar labs do not. We've found it very valuable."

STUDENT: "This man has emphysema. He's seventy-three. He's dying."

VISIT: "We are nonetheless obligated to learn all we can about his disease."

STUDENT: "But it won't help him."

VISIT: "The Respiratory Unit has multiple functions. We are at once engaged in research and therapy."

STUDENT: "Will you tell the patient that the procedure won't help him, that it's just for the sake of curiosity?"

VISIT: "I wouldn't call it curiosity."

STUDENT: "Then you have a formal experiment going? A protocol? This patient is part of a defined study series?"

VISIT: "No, but we are gathering data. All patients are available for research here."

Perhaps the most common criticism of the academic service is that "the doctors are not interested in patients, only in diseases," a harsh complaint, and an old one. Oliver Wendell Holmes said in 1867 that he did not want a researcher-clinician for his doctor: "I want a whole man for my doctor, not half a one." (As a teacher, Holmes could be brutal about academic medical instruction: "What is this stuff with which you are cramming the brains of young men who are to hold the lives of the community in their hands? Here is a man fallen in a fit; you can tell me all about the eight surfaces of the two processes of the palate-bone, but you have not had the sense to loosen the man's neck-cloth, and the old women are still calling you a fool.")

Certainly the researcher-clinician has split loyalties and conflicting interests. A GI consult who sees a patient is specifically called in to give advice about the patient's abdomen; and to some extent, the consulting physicians are more interested in the patient's stomach than the rest of him. The consequence of this may be to surround the teaching patient with many people interested in his problems, but less interested in the patient himself. The patient gets excellent but impersonal care—if that is not a contradiction in terms.

The idea that an orientation toward disease can ever lead to poor care is furiously denied by academicians. But it is disturbing to note, for instance, that Death Rounds at the MGH, which once reviewed a deceased patient's hospital course with a view to discussing whether anything more could have been done for him, are now almost entirely given over to academics: the patient's disease is discussed, not the patient. (This is only true on the medical service. Surgical Death and Complication Rounds still deal with the patient's course. In general, the surgical service is more pragmatic and less academic than the medical—a point of some friction between the two groups.)

Eventually, one comes to the conclusion that care on a teaching service is not so much better or worse as different. Some patients will benefit from these differences more than others. A patient with an obscure malady can do no better than a teaching service, where he will be fussed over, considered, and reconsidered endlessly; a patient with a common, well-understood complaint may get quicker, more practical treatment from a private doctor in a nonacademic setting.

This would seem an excellent argument for transforming the teaching hospital into a referral institution, and that is what has happened to many of them. But there are two reasons to deplore the change.

First, it means that research on the most common—and therefore, one might argue, the most important—diseases stops. This is unwise; there are many times in medical history when a researcher has "gone over old ground" and come up with something new and important. Reginald Fitz went over "perityphlitis" and came up with appendicitis, thus changing the course of surgical history.

Second, it ignores the community in which the hospital stands. The community is likely to sense this rapidly, and resent the fact that although the hospital personnel did a great job for Uncle Joe's unpronounceable Latin ailment, they could hardly be bothered with Sally's ear infection.

✠

What is the hospital's responsibility? Originally, the answer was quite clear—it was built to care for any needy person in Boston who had the initiative to seek it out. With the passage of time, its community became not the entire city, but a part of it, the so-called North End. This is a community of working-class Italians and Irishmen, with areas of considerable poverty.

But the hospital has never lost its passivity, a tradition

that can be traced all the way back to Greece. Patients are expected to come to the hospital, and not the reverse. And while the hospital will never turn anyone away from its doors, neither will it actively seek out illness in the community. Furthermore, the impact of technology over the last twenty years has been to make the hospital even more passive, as it becomes more preoccupied with acute established disease, to the almost total neglect of preventive medicine.

But the role of the hospital is going to change, as public expectations for medical care change. According to Alexander Leaf, Chief of Medicine, "For a long time —since Hippocrates—we have not attached any broader social obligation to the physician's education. You went through your training program whether in school or as an apprentice, and then you hung out your shingle and treated whoever could pay you. But now that is unacceptable to society, which is making other demands from physicians."

He says, further: "I think we have to restructure the functions of the hospital if it is to survive for the next twenty years."

Implicit in this is the notion that what the hospital now does, it does well. But it is not doing enough, and the times, indeed, are changing. To quote Galbraith, "One must either anticipate change or be its victim."

The hospital can no longer be a charitable refuge for the poor patients—the poor patient (or, rather, the patient whose bills can't be paid) is disappearing from the landscape.

The hospital can no longer act as a stronghold of technological, scientific excellence for a few patients, when the disparity between in-patient marvels and community horrors is ever-increasing.

Dr. John Knowles, director of the hospital, observes that "When I was recently the visit on the medical service, the first five patients presented to me all happened, by a curious coincidence, to have the same problem. And it serves to point up the incongruity of what we're doing here. All five were elderly, chronic alcoholics with massive GI bleeding and end-stage liver disease. All five were in coma and we were treating them vigorously, with everything medicine has to offer. They had intravenous lines, and central venous pressure catheters, and tracheostomies, and positive pressure respirators, and suction and Seng stocking tubes, and all the rest. They had house staff and students and nurses working on them around the clock. They had consultants of every shape and sort. They were running up bills of five hundred dollars a day, week after week. . . . Certainly I think they should be treated, just as I think that a large hospital like this is the place where this brand of complex medicine ought to be carried out. But you can't help reflecting, as you look at all this stainless steel and tubing and sophisticated equipment, that right outside your door there are people with TB who aren't getting antibiotics, and kids who aren't getting vaccinations, and women who aren't getting prenatal care. . . . I think we have an obligation to these other people, as well."

The hospital's new objective is to spread its resources more widely, at the expense of its traditional passivity. The first step has been to begin an ambulatory care center in Charlestown, a depressed area of 16,000 people. This sort of "satellite clinic" is widely debated in medical circles today.

Dr. Leaf: "The Charlestown project is interesting to us, to see if we can begin to restructure the way we deliver care. I hear arguments from my colleagues in the medical school, saying that no satellite clinic has ever worked. They say the research interest isn't there, the way it is in a hospital. They say you can't find doctors to work in them. Well, then, we just have to get some new physicians who see their research as working in the community, devising ways to give better care, rather than being in the hospital and doing research on, say, gastric physiology."

Certainly the academic hospitals will have to abandon what Dr. Knowles calls "the present defensive isolation . . . in a bastion of acute curative, specialized, and technical medicine." The impact of this on the inner workings of the hospital itself may be extensive, and beneficial.

✠

In 1896, the intern Harvey Cushing referred to the

MGH as "this little world of ours"—and he meant precisely that. It *was* a little world, and it *was* "ours"; it belonged to the doctors, not to the patients. Doctors were a permanent fixture in this world. The patients were transients who came and went. (Patients are well aware that the hospital is for the doctors, and not for themselves. They frequently report that they feel like "specimens in a zoo." Indeed, nearly every literate person who has recorded his experience in an academic hospital, from the late Philip Blaiberg on down, has mentioned this disturbing association.)

Initially the hospital was designed to be a little world for the patients, supplying all their needs. In those days, there were few resident physicians. But the hospital has evolved into a complete world for doctors as well. Indeed, it would be surprising if it did not, for there is one house officer for every four patients, and the house officers spend almost as much time in the hospital as the patients.

For a resident, the completeness of the little world— with its dormitories, libraries, cafeterias, coffee shops, chapel, post office, laundry, tennis and basketball courts, drugstore, magazine stand—combined with the intensity of training (the average resident spends 126 hours a week in the hospital) can have some peculiar effects. It is quite possible to forget that the hospital stands in the midst of a larger community, and that the final goal of hospitalization is reintegration of the patient into that community. In this respect, the hospital is like two other institutions which have a partially custodial function, schools and prisons. In each case, success is best measured not by the performance of the individual within the system, but after he leaves it. And in each case there is a tendency to view institutional performance as an end in itself.

This is true for both doctors and patients. The ideal of the physician-scientist, the clinician-researcher, is very much a product of academic hospital values. The educational process designed to mold this product has some paradoxical aspects. One may reasonably ask, for example, what is a medical student being trained to become?

Without doubt the answer is: a house officer in a teaching hospital. A good medical student graduates with all the necessary equipment: a background in basic science, some clinical experience, familiarity with the journals, and an academic orientation.

What, then, is a house officer being trained to become? The answer is, an academic physician specializing in acute, curative, hospital-based medicine.* This is heavily scientific and not very behavioral; it must be so. (As the visit said: "Tell me about his kidneys, not his marital troubles." And the visit was right: the hospital is geared to treat his kidneys, and not his arguments with his wife.)

But the great majority of house officers do not be-

* This same argument has been made by Peter Drucker concerning undergraduate, liberal arts colleges, where he points out that professors of English or History are not training liberal humanitarians or anything else so noble—they are training future professors of English and History.

come academic physicians, at least not full time. They go out into the community to begin, in many respects, a totally different kind of practice from any they have ever seen. They are shocked to discover that 70 per cent of their patients have no identifiable illness; they are besieged and pestered by "crocks"; they have relatively few acutely ill patients, and relatively few hospitalized patients. They are, in short, called upon to practice a great deal of behavioral art and relatively little science.

These doctors suffer from what Grossman calls "acute organically trained syndrome." The rationale for giving them the training they got, as preparation for the work they would be doing, was formerly couched as "if they can handle the problems they see in the hospital, they can handle anything." It is obviously untrue, except for those diseases that are scientifically understood and medically treatable; patients with other complaints may get a more sympathetic ear from their next-door neighbor.

Underneath it all is a sense that modern, scientific medicine can be taught, but the vague, amorphous "art" cannot be taught in the same way. This is true, but it does not mean it cannot be taught at all. Nor does it mean that simply watching the visit examine five or ten patients a week is a sufficient background in how to deal with a patient's psyche.

What a medical resident knows about science he has gotten from intensive courses, rounds, seminars, and journal reading; what he knows about behavior, psychiatry, psychology, or sociology depends on what he has managed to pick up as he goes along. This generally amounts to pitifully little.* It is hard to estimate the amount of time a doctor spends studying behavioral science during his years as a student, intern, and resident. Formal training—lectures as a student, rotations as a clinical clerk, social service and psychiatric rounds as a house officer—probably account for no more than 1 to 2 per cent of his total time; the extent of informal training is impossible to guess.

There is now a growing movement within medical education to provide more formal training in behavior, but there is also formidable opposition. As John Knowles has pointed out, medicine gained acceptance within the university as a valid discipline not because of its advances as a social science, but because of its discoveries as a natural science. For nearly a century, natural science has been the paydirt, and the behavioral art has taken a subordinate position. Reversing the trend of a century will take some doing.

Of course, the hospital has an out-patient depart-

* A student of my acquaintance, now a psychiatric resident, endeared himself to the house staff of hospitals where he was a student by doggedly asking each resident he met to define, in a simple sentence, the difference between neurosis and psychosis. He concluded that 15 per cent had some vaguely appropriate notion; the rest were appallingly wrong. The fact that a doctor does not know the difference between neurosis and psychosis does not necessarily mean he will be a poor physician; a doctor who cannot articulate these distinctions may conceivably handle them deftly in his practice. But it is a clear indication he has not had much training in behavior, and the question is whether he ought to have such training and whether his patients would benefit from the training.

ment and emergency ward, where the interface of hospital and society is more sharply seen. But the addition of community clinics, separate from the hospital, will almost certainly change the psychological set of doctors working within the physical setting of the hospital itself.

It is too early to know whether the satellite clinics are going to work. The question of physician acceptance is one problem; the question of community acceptance another. But if they do not work, something else must be found, and at this time it appears social pressures are sufficiently intense to guarantee such a search for new delivery systems.

✠

The concept of a "patient-oriented hospital" is fashionable at the moment. The phrase is widely used, though the idea is shopworn. People have recognized for a long time—at least twenty-five years—that hospitals are designed for the patient's needs only when those needs do not conflict with the doctors' convenience. Nor is there any mystery about why this is so. Whenever a new hospital is built, it is the doctors who are consulted on design requirements, not the patients.

All this has produced a great deal of talk among doctors, architects, patients, engineers, interior decorators, and innumerable other people—but very little innovation, very little experimentation. For the majority of hospitals, and the majority of new hospitals, the classic complaints still hold true:

The hospital is difficult to adapt to. It brings in individuals from outside, and plunges them into a totally new existence, with new schedules, new food, new rules, new clothing, new language, new sounds and smells, fears and rewards. For the patient entering this foreign environment, there are no guides or guidebooks available to him. A person visiting Europe can get better advance information than a person entering the "foreign country" of the hospital.

The hospital building disregards physical factors that might promote recovery. Colors are bland, but instead of being restful, are more often depressing; space is badly distributed, so that a patient may be stranded in a large room, or crowded in a small one; private and semi-private patients often feel isolated in their rooms. (A Montefiore Hospital study concluded that while families of ward patients were eager to see their relatives transferred to private rooms, the patients wanted to stay on the wards, where they would have more contact with other people.) Windows are badly placed, and the view most often shows an adjacent large hospital building or a parking lot.

The hospital makes psychological demands that may retard recovery. According to Stanley King, these include dependence and compliance with hospital routine; a de-emphasis on external power and prestige; tolerance for pain and suffering; and the expectation that a patient will want to get well. These can easily work at cross-purposes. For example, a proudly self-reliant man may find his passive role as threatening as his illness. Or a person may become so dependent, and regress so far toward a childlike state, that he becomes more petty, complaining, and intolerant of pain than he would be otherwise. Or he may find his dependent role so satisfying that he loses his desire to get well.

One may immediately object that despite all this, the majority of patients adjust well to the hospital, recover, and go home. That is true, but as an argument it is a little like saying that the world got on perfectly well without electricity, which is also true.

But assuming these complaints have validity—assuming that patients would really recover more swiftly in a better designed environment—how should the new environment be designed? There is a spectrum of proposals, ranging from minor adjustments to quite radical innovations.

Perhaps the most radical, and the most interesting, comes from a simple observation: the modern hospital is best suited to a severely ill person. These people are most tolerant of hospital routine and its indignities, irritants, and difficulties.

On the other hand, persons recovering frequently become less tolerant as their physical condition improves. The phenomenon is so well known that doctors notice when a previously compliant patient begins to grumble about the food or the noise at night. These gripes are interpreted as a sure sign the patient is improving. Related to this is the so-called "lipstick sign," referring to

216

the fact that as women begin to feel better, they start wearing lipstick and combing their hair in the morning. Essentially, all this means that the patients are acting in ways not demanded by the environment (lipstick) or else positively condemned by the environment (griping). Such activities are more appropriate to the outside world, and they are a signal that the patient, in his own mind, is preparing to leave the hospital for the outside.

How can one capitalize on this? At present, not at all. This is because, at the present time, patients are assigned to different parts of the hospital on the basis of only three criteria—financial resources, sex, and anticipated therapy. No other attribute of the patient matters, not even diagnosis. (Patients with ulcers, pancreatitis, or cancer, for example, will be assigned to medical or surgical floors depending on whether their treatment calls for operation or not.)

The various floors of the hospital operate with their own nurses, their own visits, their own house staff, their own stocks of supplies. This is the arrangement found in most American hospitals, and as a way of structuring, it has distinct advantages. For many years, it was thought to be the best way of matching the patient to the facilities he would most need.

However, each of the three criteria—sex, money, and therapy—has come under attack. Money, because third-party payment has made financial structuring obsolete; sex, because if everyone is in private or semi-private rooms, segregation by whole floors becomes unnecessary.

Anticipated therapy has also been questioned. Some even argue that the distinction between surgical and medical patients be abandoned in favor of distinctions based on severity of illness, and the need for close medical and nursing attention.

Under this system, medical and surgical patients would be intermixed in units that differed in the degree of care they provided—intensive care, recuperative care, minimal care, and so on. Patients would be moved about in the hospital as their illness became greater or less.

Some clear psychological benefits for patients are apparent. As they became healthier, they would be moved to new areas of the hospital, where they would be encouraged to be more self-sufficient, to wear their own clothes, to look after themselves, to go down to the cafeteria and get their own food, and so on. They would, at every point, be surrounded by patients of equal severity of illness. Their dependency needs would be fulfilled in a graded way, since the hospital was providing a spectrum of care and close attention.

To a degree, the hospital already does this, with its recovery rooms and intensive-care units.* But more could be done—and, indeed, one can predict that more will almost certainly be done in this direction. This will happen not because the hospital is preoccupied with the

* The hospital already has intensive-care units for respiratory care, cardiac care, neurological care, surgical care, medical care, transplantation patients, pediatric patients, and burns patients.

patient's psyche—it is not—but rather because graded care is economically more efficient. At the present time 30 per cent of the cost of a room goes to nursing care. For the average MGH hospital room, this amounts to some $22 a day. Although the percentage cost may not rise in the future, the absolute cost will. Ultimately it will be necessary to give patients no more nursing care than they really need; the present inefficiency in personnel use will become too costly to continue.

Among physicians, a restructuring could be more efficient as well. Consider anesthetists: in the last decade, they have emerged as the experts in the support of vital functions. They are called for every cardiac and respiratory arrest; they know more about drugs than anyone else; they are expert in the use of respirators. Most physicians would agree it is handy to have an anesthetist around any intensive-care unit, but at present the anesthetists are dispersed throughout the hospital. By restructuring on the basis of severity of illness, one important resource, anesthetists, would be made more available to patients who need them.

Indeed, "human resources" are just one argument for restructuring. Hardware and technology resources represent another. For example, the kind of electronic and mechanical equipment required for a patient with a heart attack and for a post-operative cardiac patient is very similar. As time goes on, and larger and more all-inclusive machines become available, it will be increasingly advantageous to bring patients with similar technological requirements together, so that they may share certain large machine capabilities and so that medical personnel trained in the use of these machines can be centralized.

The bringing together of patients, personnel, and hardware has certainly been valuable in cardiac intensive care units; in some units immediate mortality from myocardial infarction has been cut as much as 30 per cent. We are already seeing a proliferation of these specialized units, and we will certainly see more—and from there it is only a small step to complete reordering of the hospital along new lines.

AFTERWORD

Although it comes from an ancient tradition, the modern hospital, in fully recognizable form, is less than fifty years old.

At most it will last, in fully recognizable form, another decade or so. But by then, almost surely, what is different from the present will overshadow what is similar. And we may expect these changes to represent more than improved technology and differently trained personnel. For there will certainly be a change in the function of hospitals, just as there has been a change in function during the past half century.

During that period, the hospital evolved into a positive, curative agency specializing in highly technical, complex medical procedures. Very likely the hospital will continue to function in this capacity. But it will abandon certain other functions in the process. It will cease to be a convalescent facility, for example, as more specialized convalescent homes appear. It will curtail its in-patient diagnostic work to that which absolutely requires hospitalization. Its custodial function—whether represented by a young couple "dumping" grandpa for the weekend, so that they can have a few days to themselves, or by the admission of alcoholics and derelicts who would otherwise have nowhere to go—has already been reduced and will soon be eliminated. One can say this with some confidence because in every case the rationale is economic, not philosophical. Hospitals are becoming so expensive that financial considerations will soon become the paramount determinant of function.

Less certain are those new tasks and responsibilities that the hospital will assume in the future. Here, the pressures are largely social, and their manifestations not easily anticipated. Perhaps the clearest—and most general—trend is the hospital's notion of an extended responsibility, which goes beyond the confines of its walls. A teaching hospital such as the Massachusetts General now sees its job as dealing both with the hospital patients, and with the surrounding community. It defines this new role in two ways: discovering those patients who need hospitalization but are not receiving it, and treating other patients so that future hospitalizations will be prevented.

But the hospital is going further. It is spreading its

research and its knowledge beyond the local community to a broader population. In the past, it did this in the form of research papers printed in scientific journals. That form persists, but more directly the hospital now uses television and computer programs to disseminate its knowledge and its resources.

For the patient, something rather paradoxical is happening. Broadly speaking, the whole thrust of enlightened medical thinking is directed toward getting more care to more people. The problem is as enormous and as important as curing any specific disease process. In examining the situation, both doctors and patients express the fear that the individual may cease to be treated as a person, that he may become merged into some faceless, very lonely crowd. Yet at the same time, the hospitals, which have traditionally been the most impersonal elements in any health-care system, are more concerned than ever about tailoring the hospital so it treats every patient individually.

For medical education, the impact of changes in hospital function may be considerable. For the last half century, medical education has been almost exclusively in-patient education—the emphasis has been upon care of the patient who is in the hospital and not outside it. But as the hospital reaches outside its walls, so will medical education.

There is another point about medical education, not often considered in formal discussions. It is a problem, a fact of medical life, which can be dated quite precisely in terms of origin: it began in 1923, with Banting and Best. The discovery of insulin by these workers led directly to the first chronic therapy of complexity and seriousness, where administration lay in the hands of the patient. Prior to that time, there were indeed chronic medications—such as digitalis for heart failure or colchicine for gout—but a patient taking such medications did not need to be terribly careful about it or terribly knowledgeable about his disease process. That is to say, if he took his medicines irregularly, he developed medical difficulties fairly slowly, or else he developed difficulties that were not life-threatening.

Insulin was different. A patient had to be careful or he might die in a matter of hours. And since insulin there has come a whole range of chronic therapies that are equally complex and serious, and that require a knowledgeable, responsible patient.

Partly in response to these demands, partly as a consequence of better education, patients are more knowledgeable about medicine than ever before. Only the most insecure and unintelligent physicians wish to keep patients from becoming even more knowledgeable.

And when one considers a medical institution, such as the hospital, the importance of a knowledgeable public becomes still clearer. Hospitals are now changing. They will change more, and faster, in the future. Much of that change will be a response to social pressure, a demand for services and facilities. It is vital that this demand be intelligent, and informed.

Glossary &

Bibliography

Glossary

abrasions Scrapes.

acidosis Excessive acidity in the blood.

acute In medical reference, meaning of short duration. There is no connotation of severity. The opposite of an acute illness is a chronic illness.

ampoule A drug container, usually made of glass.

amylase An enzyme produced in the pancreas and found in elevated blood concentration when the pancreas is diseased.

amyloidosis A disease characterized by deposits of amyloid in various tissues. Amyloid is a protein substance.

angiogram An X-ray study of blood vessels.

arrhythmia Irregular heartbeat.

barium A metallic element. Barium sulfate, a salt, is opaque to X rays and is not absorbed by the gastrointestinal tract. When a liquid suspension of barium sulfate is swallowed by the patient, the stomach and intestine are outlined in white on X rays and can be better studied.

bilirubin A golden pigment formed when the hemoglobin in red blood cells is broken down. Bilirubin is normally excreted by the body; in various disease states it can accumulate, causing jaundice (*q.v.*).

biopsy Removal of a sample of living tissue for examination.

blood pressure Expressed in millimeters of mercury, this is generally the pressure within the brachial artery of the arm. Blood pressure is expressed as a fraction, such as $120/80$. The first figure is known as systolic blood pressure, and represents the peak pressure inside the artery corresponding to each contraction of the heart. The smaller figure is known as diastolic blood pressure, and represents the pressure inside the artery between contractions.

blood sugar Blood normally contains a certain amount of sugar, but the amount can be increased in disease states such as diabetes.

bone marrow aspiration Removal of some bone marrow by suction through a needle.

catheter A hollow cylinder of metal, rubber, or plastic designed to be passed through any of several body channels, such as the arteries, veins, or the urinary system.

catheterize To pass a catheter through a body channel.

celiac angiogram An X-ray study of blood vessels which supply abdominal organs, that is, of the so-called celiac arteries.

cerebrospinal fluid The fluid which bathes the brain and spinal cord.

cirrhosis From the Greek for "tawny," and the early observation that scarred organs became yellowish in appearance. The term refers to destruction of parts of an organ and replacement of the damaged areas by fibrous scar tissue. One can speak of cirrhosis of breasts, kidney, or lung, but the term usually refers to scarring of the liver, following damage from alcohol or other causes.

CPK Creatinine phosphokinase, an enzyme. When the concentration of this enzyme in the blood is increased, it suggests tissue damage, particularly heart muscle damage.

CSF Cerebrospinal fluid (*q.v.*).

digitalis A drug to improve the strength of heart muscle.

disseminated cancer Widespread or metastatic (*q.v.*).

diuretic A drug that promotes excretion of urine.

diverticulitis Inflammation of a diverticulum, generally the tiny diverticula of the lower intestine.

diverticulum Literally a pouch opening out from some hollow organ, such as the gut or bladder.

edema Accumulation of excessive fluid in tissues; dropsy. It can be observed in a wide range of disease states.

electrocardiogram A graphic record of the electrical activity of the heart, revealing information about the rhythm, the electrical conduction within the heart, the health and thickness of heart muscle, and so on.

encephalitis Inflammation of the brain.

glomerulonephritis Inflammation of the kidney; specifically, of a part of the kidney known as the glomerulus.

guarding In medical reference, it refers to a patient's tensing his muscles in a painful area when he is touched there.

hematocrit A centrifuge for separating cells from the liquid portion of the blood. In medicalese, the volume percentage of red cells to fluid in blood. Normally 40 to 45 per cent.

hepatitis Inflammation of the liver, usually caused by a virus.

idiopathic Of unknown origin.

IVP Intravenous pyelogram, an X-ray study of kidneys made while they excrete a special dye.

jaundice A yellow staining of skin and eyes, from accumulation of bilirubin (*q.v.*) in the body.

lacerations Cuts.

LDH Lactic dehydrogenase, an enzyme. Blood levels are increased with tissue destruction in various organs.

lumbar puncture Passage of a needle between lumbar vertebrae in the lower spine, in order to enter the spinal canal and remove for analysis some of the fluid that bathes the brain and spinal cord.

metastatic cancer Cancer that has spread throughout the body to distant sites.

myocardial infarction Heart attack.

morphology Physical appearance.

obtunded Literally blunted, in medical reference to demonstrate decreased mental alertness and acuity.

pancreatitis Inflammation of the pancreas.

pathological Diseased, abnormal.

platelet A small, flat, plate-like cell in the blood that aids in clotting.

platelet count A count of such cells.

prognosis Foretelling of the outcome of a disease.

reticulocyte An immature blood cell.

reticulocyte count A counting of the number of immature red cells in circulation. Normally only a small percentage of red cells are immature; if the bone marrow is making more blood, the number of reticulocytes in circulation will increase.

sequestered Hidden.

SGOT Serum glutamic oxaloacetic transaminase, an enzyme. When present in elevated concentrations in blood, it implies tissue damage.

stenosis Narrowing of any canal or aperture, such as aortic stenosis, narrowing of the aortic valve of the heart.

sternum Breastbone.

steroids A class of chemical agents with a characteristic ring structure that are produced within the body (as well as artificially). Many sex hormones are steroids. Corticosteroids, which are produced in the cortex of the adrenal glands, have the power to suppress inflammation and the immune response.

tap As in thoracic or abdominal tap, medicalese for passage of a needle into the chest or abdomen to drain off ("tap") fluid inside; centesis.

toxin Poison.

triage officer An emergency-ward physician who decides which patient requires treatment first.

ventricles The paired lower chambers of the heart.

Bibliography: REFERENCES

All cited sources are listed below,
as well as others which provide
the general background for the book

"Annual Report of Vital Statistics of Massachusetts, 1933–1953."

"Annual Reports, Massachusetts General Hospital, 1821–1967."

Aub, J. C., *et al: Management of the Cocoanut Grove Burns at the Massachusetts General Hospital.* Philadelphia: Lippincott; 1943.

Bowditch, N. I.: *History of the Massachusetts General Hospital, 1810–1872.* Boston: Griffith-Stillings; 1872.

Burrage, W. L.: *A History of the Massachusetts Medical Society, 1781–1922.* Norwood, Massachusetts: Privately Printed; 1923.

Churchill, E. D.: *At Work in the Vineyards of Surgery; the Reminiscences of J. Collins Warren, 1842–1927.* Edited with appendices, notes, and comments by E. D. Churchill. Cambridge: Harvard University Press; 1958.

"Commonwealth of Massachusetts, Registration Report, 1883–1903."

Faxon, N. W.: *The Massachusetts General Hospital, 1935–1955.* Cambridge: Harvard University Press; 1959.

Garland, J. E.: *Every Man Our Neighbor, A Brief History of the Massachusetts General Hospital, 1811–1961.* Boston: Little, Brown; 1961.

Harrington, T. F.: *The Harvard Medical School, 1872–1905, a History, Narrative and Documentary.* Edited in three volumes by J. G. Mumford. New York: Lewis; 1905.

"Massachusetts General Hospital, Directions as to the Diet of Patients." Boston: Privately Printed; 1850.

Massachusetts General Hospital Memorial and Historical Volume (together with proceedings of the Centennial of the opening of the Hospital). Boston: Griffith-Stillings; 1921.

Massachusetts General Hospital, Rules Concerning the Decease of a Patient. Boston: Privately Printed; 1850.

Massachusetts General Hospital, Rules for House Officers. Boston: Privately Printed; 1850.

Means, J. H.: *Ward 4, The Mallinkrockdt Research Ward of the Massachusetts General Hospital.* Cambridge: Harvard University Press; 1958.

Myers, G. W.: *History of the Massachusetts General Hospital, 1872–1900.* Boston: Griffith-Stillings; 1929.

Washburn, F. A.: *The Massachusetts General Hospital. Its Development 1900–1935.* Boston: Houghton Mifflin; 1939.

MEDICAL HISTORY

Fulton, J. F.: *Harvey Cushing, A Biography.* Springfield, Illinois: Thomas; 1946.

Garrison, F. H.: *Contributions to the History of Medicine.* New York: Hafner; 1966.

Inglis, B.: *A History of Medicine.* New York: World; 1965.

Major, J. H.: *Classic Descriptions of Disease.* Third Edition. Springfield, Illinois: Thomas; 1945.

Moore, F. D.: *The Gastrointestinal Tract: Surgery.* Edited by Richard Warren. Philadelphia: Saunders; 1963.

Richardson, R. G.: *The Surgeon's Tale.* London: Allen and Unwin; 1958.

Riesman, D.: *The Story of Medicine in the Middle Ages.* New York: Hoeber; 1935.

Rogers, F. B.: *A Syllabus of Medical History.* Boston: Little, Brown; 1962.

Roueché, B.: *Curiosities of Medicine.* Boston: Little, Brown; 1958.

Sigerist, H.: *A History of Medicine.* Oxford: Oxford University Press; 1951.

Henry E. Sigerist on the History of Medicine. Edited by Felix Martí-Ibañez. New York: MD Publications; 1960.

COMMENTARY

Barnett, G. O.: "Computers in Patient Care." *New England Journal of Medicine,* 279 (1968), pp. 1314–18.

Beeson, P. B.: "Review of Sickness and Society." *Yale Journal of Biology and Medicine,* 41 (1968), pp. 226–41.

Bell, D.: *Toward the Year 2000: Work in Progress.* Edited by Daniel Bell. Boston: Beacon; 1969.

Bellin, S. S., *et al:* "Impact of Ambulatory Health Care Services on the Demand for Hospital Beds." *New England Journal of Medicine,* 280 (1969), pp. 808–12.

Burling, T., *et al: The Give and Take in Hospitals.* New York: Putnam's; 1956.

Burnet, F. M.: *The Integrity of the Body.* Cambridge: Harvard University Press; 1963.

Charnley, J., *et al:* "Penetration of Gown Material by Organisms from the Surgeon's Body." *Lancet* 1 (1969), pp. 172–3.

Cheever, D.: "The Turn of the Century—and After." *New England Journal of Medicine,* 222 (1940), pp. 1–11.

Coleman, J. S.: *Medical Innovation: A Diffusion Study.* Indianapolis: Bobbs-Merrill; 1961.

Dombal, F. T., *et al:* "A Computer-Assisted System for Learning Clinical Diagnosis." *Lancet* 1 (1969), pp. 145–8.

Dubos, R.: *Man Adapting.* New Haven: Yale University Press; 1965.

——: *Mirage of Health.* New York: Harper; 1959.

Duff, R. S., *et al: Sickness and Society.* New York: Harper and Row; 1968.

Ebert, R. H.: *Medical Education and the University: Views of Medical Education.* Edited by J. H. Knowles. Cambridge: Harvard University Press; 1967.

——: *The Dilemma of Medical Teaching in an Affluent Society: The Teaching Hospital.* Edited by J. H. Knowles. Cambridge: Harvard University Press; 1966.

237

Gell, P. G. H., *et al: Clinical Aspects of Immunology.* Philadelphia: Davis; 1962.

Hartog, J. de: *The Hospital.* New York: Atheneum; 1964.

Henderson, L. J.: *The Study of Man.* Philadelphia: University of Pennsylvania Press; 1941.

Holmes, O. W.: *Medical Essays.* Boston: Houghton Mifflin; 1882.

King, S. H.: *Perception of Illness and Medical Practice.* New York: Russell Sage; 1962.

Kissick, W. L.: "Planning, Programming and Budgeting in Health." *Medical Care,* 5 (1967), pp. 201–20.

Knowles, J. H.: *Medical Education and the Rationalization of Health Services: Views of Medical Education and Medical Care.* Edited by J. H. Knowles. Cambridge: Harvard University Press; 1968.

——: *Medical School, Teaching Hospital, and Social Responsibility: The Teaching Hospital.* Edited by J. H. Knowles. Cambridge: Harvard University Press; 1966.

——: "The Balanced Biology of the Teaching Hospital." *New England Journal of Medicine,* 269 (1963), pp. 401–6, 450–5.

——: *The Teaching Hospital: Historical Perspective and a Contemporary View: Hospitals, Doctors, and the Public Interest.* Edited by J. H. Knowles. Cambridge: Harvard University Press; 1965.

Lasagna, L.: *Life, Death and the Doctor.* New York: Alfred A. Knopf; 1968.

Lewis, C. E., *et al:* "Activities, Events and Outcomes in Ambulatory Patient Care." *New England Journal of Medicine,* 280 (1969), pp. 645–49.

Linn, B. S.: "Statistics, Computers, and Clinical Judgement." *Lancet* 2 (1968), pp. 48–50.

Means, J. H.: "Homo Medicus Americanus." *Daedalus,* 92 (1963), pp. 701–22.

Mechanic, D.: *Medical Sociology.* New York: The Free Press; 1968.

Merton, R. K., *et al: The Student-Physician.* Cambridge: Harvard University Press; 1957.

COMMENTARY

MRC Report: "Aseptic Methods in the Operating Suite." *Lancet* 1 (1969), pp. 705–10, 763–8, 831–7.

Neurath, P. W. *et al*: "Design of a Computer System to Assist in Differential Preoperative Diagnosis for Pelvic Surgery." *New England Journal of Medicine*, 280 (1969), pp. 785–90.

Orwell, G.: "How the Poor Die." *Shooting an Elephant and Other Essays*. New York: Harcourt, Brace; 1950.

Piel, G.: *Science in the Cause of Man*. New York: Alfred A. Knopf; 1961.

Platt, R.: *The New Medicine and Its Responsibilities: The Humanist Frame*. Edited by J. Huxley. London: Allen and Unwin; 1961.

Powledge, F.: "What Will the Doctors Do for Jean Paul Getty that they won't do for you?" *Esquire* (October 1968).

Russell, P. S.: *Surgery in a Time of Change: The Teaching Hospital*. Edited by J. H. Knowles. Cambridge: Harvard University Press; 1966.

Rutstein, D. D.: *The Company Revolution in Medicine*. Cambridge: MIT Press; 1968.

Schuck, H., *et al*: *Nobel, The Man and His Prizes*. New York: Elsevier Publishing Company; 1962.

Shattuck, F. C.: "The Science and Art of Medicine in Some of Their Aspects." *Boston Medical and Surgical Journal*, 157 (1907), pp. 63–7.

Smith, H. L., *et al*: *Patients, Physicians and Illness*. Glencoe, Illinois: The Free Press; 1958.

Weil, A. T.: "Conversations with a Mechanical Psychiatrist." *Harvard Review*, No. 3 (1965), pp. 68–74.